Quick Cooking for
Diabetes

Quick Cooking for
Diabetes

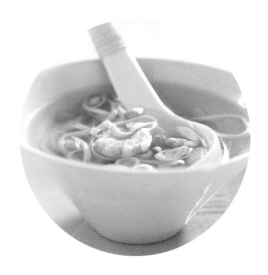

great tasting food in 30 minutes or less

Louise Blair & Norma McGough

hamlyn

Diabetes UK is the charity for people with diabetes. It represents their interests by campaigning for better standards of care and by funding research to find a cure for diabetes and improve treatments. It offers advice and support on all aspects of the condition through its many books and leaflets and the internet. There is a confidential careline, operated by fully trained counsellors, for general enquiries from people with diabetes, their carers and healthcare professionals.

For further information please see www.diabetes.org.uk or contact us at:

10 Parkway
London NW1 7AA
Tel: 020 7323 1531
Fax: 020 7637 3644
Email: info@diabetes.org.uk

First published in Great Britain in 2002 by Hamlyn
an imprint of Octopus Publishing Group Limited
2–4 Heron Quays
London E14 4JP

Copyright © 2002 Octopus Publishing Group Limited

ISBN 0600 60438 1

British Library Cataloguing-in-Publication Data
A catalogue record for this book is available from the British Library

Printed and bound in China
10 9 8 7 6 5 4 3 2 1

The publisher has taken all reasonable care in the preparation of this book but the information it contains is not intended to take the place of treatment by a qualified medical practitioner.

NOTES
Both metric and imperial measurements are given for the recipes. Use one set of measures only, not a mixture of both.

Ovens should be preheated to the specified temperature. If using a fan-assisted oven, follow the manufacturer's instructions for adjusting the time and temperature. Grills should also be preheated.

A few recipes include nuts and nut derivatives. Anyone with a known nut allergy must avoid these.

Free-range medium eggs should be used unless otherwise stated. The Department of Health advises that eggs should not be consumed raw. It is prudent for more vulnerable people such as pregnant and nursing mothers, invalids, the elderly, babies and young children to avoid uncooked or lightly cooked dishes made with eggs.

Meat and poultry should be cooked thoroughly. To test if poultry is cooked, pierce the flesh through the thickest part with a skewer or fork – the juices should run clear, never pink or red.

All the recipes in this book have been analysed by a State Registered Dietitian. The analysis refers to each serving.

All recipes serve 4

Contents

1 introduction   6

what is diabetes?   8

• The main types of diabetes • Managing your diabetes

• Managing your weight • Hypoglycaemia

nutrition and diabetes   12

• Healthy eating guidelines for people with diabetes • Food groups

• The glycaemic index • Sample menus

living with diabetes   22

• Healthy cooking • Reducing your fat intake • Top 10 shopping tips

• Understanding food labels • Eating out

2 rice, pasta and other grains   26

A selection of recipes using cereals and grains as the basis for complete meals

3 beans, seeds and pulses   52

Great ideas for alternatives to meat. Peas, beans and pulses

play an important part in lowering the glycaemic index in meals

4 eat more potatoes   72

Balanced meals based on potatoes. The recipes in this chapter

dispel the myth that potatoes are fattening and therefore taboo

5 extra fruit and vegetables   92

Side dishes to complement main meals and increase fruit and vegetable

intake, as well as recipes that serve as a meal in themselves

6 bread as a basis   118

Bread-based recipes that show how this staple food can be used to

bump up carbohydrate at any time of the day

Glossary   140

Index   142

Acknowledgements   144

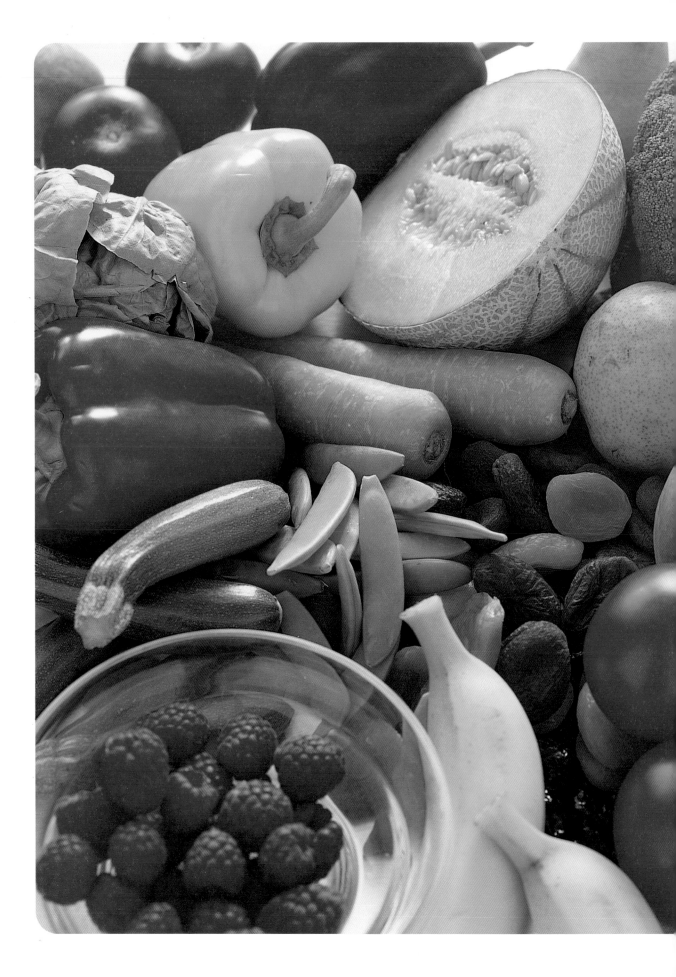

Introduction

If you have diabetes, you might think that there are certain foods that you can't eat, or that you can't enjoy social occasions in the same way as someone who doesn't have diabetes. This is not necessarily the case: in *Quick Cooking for Diabetes* you will learn how to make changes to your choice of food, your eating habits and cooking, to help you manage your diabetes more effectively and live life to the full.

The recipes in *Quick Cooking for Diabetes* have been allocated their appropriate glycaemic index – this is a way of ranking foods containing carbohydrate according to their effect on blood glucose levels. If you have diabetes, combining foods with a low glycaemic index with main meals can help to control blood glucose levels.

Diet makes all the difference to the long-term health of someone with diabetes. If you have diabetes you should reduce your intake of fat, particularly saturated or animal fat, base your meals and snacks on carbohydrate foods like bread and pasta and also eat plenty of fruit and vegetables. Salt and sugar should be used in only minimal amounts.

Eating for good health is about matching your intake of food to your body's needs and keeping your weight at a healthy level. It is also about understanding how to balance food choices, so that you can enjoy eating without feeling guilty. Even high-fat, high-sugar foods can be incorporated into your diet plan, if you know how.

what is diabetes?

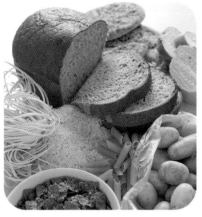

Diabetes is a common condition in which the glucose (sugar) level in the blood is too high. Normally, the level of glucose in the blood is controlled by a hormone called insulin, which is produced by the pancreas. Insulin enables the glucose to enter various cells in the body, where it is used to fuel the body's energy requirements. In the case of someone with diabetes, the body doesn't produce any or enough insulin to regulate the glucose, or the insulin that it does produce does not do the job properly. As a result, the glucose is unable to get into the cells where it is required to provide energy and instead remains in the bloodstream at high levels. Glucose comes from the digestion of starchy foods such as bread and pasta, from sugar and other sweet foods, and it is also made in the liver.

The number of cases of diabetes is increasing. It is currently estimated that 150 million people worldwide suffer from diabetes.

Diabetes is a genetic condition, which means that it tends to run in families. In addition, scientists are uncertain as to whether any environmental factors may also play a part in the development of diabetes.

It is currently estimated that 150 million of the world's population have diabetes. This is expected to rise to 300 million by the year 2025. Diabetes is more common among certain ethnic groups, particularly Asian and African-Caribbean populations. Currently about 3 per cent of people in the UK are known to have diabetes (about 1.4 million people) and for every person diagnosed with diabetes, there is probably another person who does not know they have the condition. In the US, nearly 16 million people (almost 6 per cent of the population) have diabetes, of whom 5 million are unaware that they have it. Although diabetes can occur at any age, it is rare in young children and becomes more common as people get older.

The main types of diabetes

There are two main types of diabetes: *Type 1* and *Type 2*.

◗ *Type 1*, or insulin dependent, diabetes develops when the body stops producing insulin because the cells in the pancreas that make it have been destroyed. It usually appears before the age of 40 and is treated by insulin injections and diet.

◗ *Type 2* diabetes, or non insulin dependent diabetes, is the most common type of diabetes. It develops when the body can still produce insulin, but not enough for its needs, or when the insulin that it does produce does not work properly. It usually appears in people over the age of 40 and may be treated by diet alone, or by diet in conjunction with tablets or insulin injections. People who are overweight are more likely to develop Type 2 diabetes and at least 80 per cent of people diagnosed with Type 2 diabetes have a weight problem.

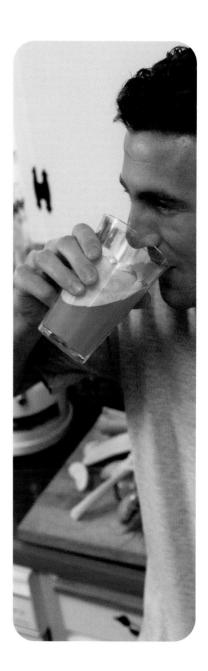

The main symptoms of untreated diabetes are increased thirst, frequently passing large amounts of urine, extreme tiredness, weight loss, genital itching and blurred vision.

Managing your diabetes

Managing your diabetes is simply about everyday control – keeping your blood glucose levels as close to normal as you can, while still maintaining a normal lifestyle. Blood glucose levels are measured in millimols per litre of blood and your doctor or diabetes nurse will be able to advise you on the levels that are best for you.

Essentially, blood glucose levels can be controlled by sticking to sensible eating habits and choosing the best foods for your body's system, together with following a healthy lifestyle that involves exercise and not smoking. These factors, in conjunction with diabetes medication if necessary, will help to protect against the long-term complications of diabetes. These can include damage to the eyes, kidneys, nerves, heart and major arteries.

Managing your weight

What you eat directly affects your weight and your blood glucose levels. It can also influence the amount of fat in your blood. If you are overweight, losing weight will help you control your diabetes. Talk to your doctor if you are not sure how much you need to lose or how to lose it. You should also discuss any dietary changes, as you may need to adjust your medication at the same time. If you are overweight, even losing just 2.5kg (5lb) and keeping it off will be beneficial to your health. Losing weight:

- Helps to control blood glucose levels by reducing the body's resistance to insulin
- Helps lower blood fats like cholesterol
- Lowers blood pressure
- Reduces the risk of heart disease and stroke

Cutting down and being more active

It is important to monitor your diabetes carefully when making changes to your diet. Cutting down on snacks or simply choosing low-fat foods like fruit instead of biscuits may be all that is required to lose weight. Or you may need to go a step further and cut down on the amount of food you normally eat at a meal, in particular cutting down on fatty foods in your diet. Eating more fruit and vegetables at meal times can help reduce your calorie intake, while still providing the volume of food you are used to eating.

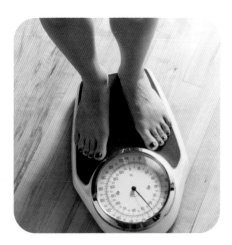

If you have diabetes you should have regular check-ups with your doctor or diabetes nurse to make sure that your diabetes is under control, and to screen for any of the complications associated with diabetes.

Becoming more active will also help you to lose weight, as well as improve your sensitivity to insulin and your general health and fitness. Remember that making gradual lifestyle changes that you can maintain in the long term will be more successful than trying to implement sudden and radical new changes. A combination of increased exercise and fewer calories is the best way to lose weight.

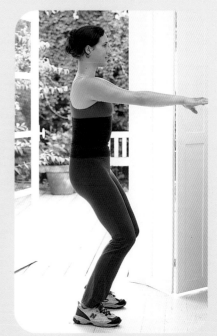

Hypoglycaemia

If you have diabetes it is important to keep your blood glucose levels fairly stable in order to minimize the risk of developing any of the long-term complications of diabetes (see page 9). 'Hypo' (short for hypoglycaemia) is a term used to describe a low blood glucose level. A hypo can be unpleasant and is more likely to happen when you are treated with insulin, but can also happen if you take certain diabetes tablets.

What causes a hypo?

However well controlled your diabetes is, you may still experience a hypo because of a late or missed meal or too little carbohydrate at a meal. Other reasons for having hypoglycaemia may include having too much insulin or medication, or drinking excess alcohol or having alcohol without food. Alcohol inhibits glucose production by the liver and in this way can lower blood glucose levels. Changing medication or undertaking unusually strenuous activity without having additional carbohydrate may also trigger a hypo, because exercise also lowers blood glucose levels.

Treating a hypo

If you identify the symptoms of a hypo (see box, top right), take some form of sugar immediately in order to make sure your blood glucose level rises and returns to normal. Sugar in the form of a sugary soft drink or four or five glucose sweets should provide enough to treat the symptoms, but it is important to make sure that your blood glucose levels get back to normal before you do anything else. You should also have a meal or snack containing some sort of carbohydrate food, such as bread, pasta or cereal, immediately after you have treated your hypo, to ensure that your glucose level is safe.

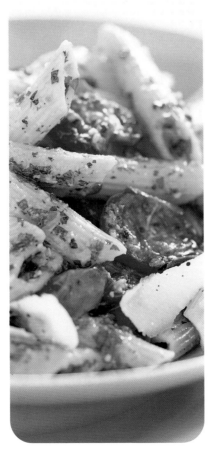

Hypo symptoms

The most common symptoms of hypoglycaemia are:

- Sweating
- Trembling
- Feeling hungry
- Anxiety and irritability
- Fast pulse and palpitations
- Blurred vision
- Tingling lips
- Going pale

nutrition and diabetes

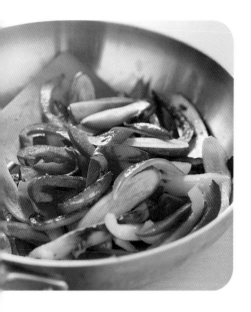

As more and more information is collected from research into diabetes, the dietary guidelines for people with diabetes have tended to change in emphasis. If you are diagnosed with diabetes, you should aim to shift the balance of your diet (see the guidelines, opposite) so as to control your blood glucose levels and help you manage your condition more easily. However, you should consider the guidelines as goals that you move towards rather than rigid targets. Start by assessing your current eating habits and consider any changes that you need to make to your usual diet, your food choices or meal planning in the context of a framework, rather than as a set of rules that can never be broken. Establishing long-term healthy eating habits can also help you reach personal targets such as your ideal weight and good cholesterol and blood pressure levels. The goals you set for yourself do not have to seem impossible. They can be as simple and straightforward as eating a piece of fruit instead of a biscuit as a snack, adding salad or vegetables to your main meal, or using pasta or pulses a couple of times a week. The main areas to consider are reducing fat and salt intake, eating more starchy carbohydrate foods, as well as fruits, vegetables and pulses, and enjoying a good variety of foods – and recipes.

In the past, a restricted carbohydrate diet and, in particular, a restricted sugar intake was considered the best way to control diabetes. As a result, many people still believe that if you have diabetes you have to stick to a rigid diet and cut out foods such as cakes and puddings. This is not the case at all and, whatever your individual dietary needs, the meals you make for yourself can be quite delicious and just as suitable for all your family and friends as well. In the same way, you don't have to miss out on special occasions – it is simply more important to get it right most of the time.

Anyone diagnosed with diabetes should see a State Registered Dietitian through their doctor or hospital. A dietitian will provide specific dietary advice and help you work out individual targets based on your particular needs and lifestyle, enabling you to feel more in control of your diabetes.

It is not necessarily the case that if you have diabetes you have to stick to a rigid diet and cut out foods such as cakes and puddings. You should still be able to enjoy a wide variety of different foods as part of a balanced diet.

Healthy eating guidelines for people with diabetes

Weight management

This is an essential aspect of diabetes care. Being overweight makes it more difficult for you to control your blood glucose levels, your blood cholesterol levels and your blood pressure. So, it is important to try to get to the weight that is right for you and retain it. If you need to lose weight, aim for a gradual weight loss that you can maintain in the long term.

Have regular meals

Eat regularly throughout the day and base your meals on starchy carbohydrate foods such as bread, potatoes, rice, pasta and cereals. If your weight is at a healthy level, this will also help to keep your blood glucose levels stable and within a reasonable range. Go a step further and choose or incorporate carbohydrate foods with a low glycaemic index (see page 17). These include pasta, rye bread, wholegrain cereals, fruits and pulses.

Cut down on saturated fat

Eat fewer foods that are rich in saturated fat, such as fatty meats, butter, cheese, cream and full-fat dairy foods (full-cream milk). Instead of butter, choose reduced- or low-fat spreads high in unsaturated fat (olive oil, rapeseed oil and sunflower oil), opt for light crème fraîche instead of double cream and use skimmed or semi-skimmed milk.

Cut down on salt

Try not to add salt to your food – use subtle flavourings such as herbs and spices instead. Look for reduced-sodium (salt) foods when buying bread and canned foods, and avoid too many salted snacks such as crisps and nuts.

Eat more fruit, vegetables and pulses

You should aim to eat five portions of fruit, vegetables and pulses every day. This will help to lower the glycaemic index of your diet, as well as balance your meals and provide you with a source of antioxidant vitamins and minerals. It will also help you to shift the balance of what you eat, if you are trying to lose weight. Eat the same volume of food each day as you do now, but a greater proportion of fruit and vegetables, and you will end up eating a much healthier diet.

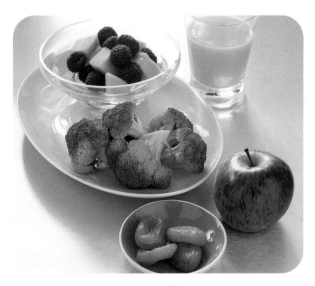

Limit your intake of sugary foods

Avoid sweets, chocolates and sugary drinks. Your diet does not have to be sugar free, but restrict sugar, fat and calories if you are trying to lose weight.

Keep to safe drinking limits

This means a maximum of two units per day for women and three units per day for men. (One unit is the equivalent of one glass of wine, one measure of a spirit and half a pint of beer, cider or lager.) Never drink on an empty stomach as alcohol can bring on a 'hypo' (see page 11) if you are on insulin injections or certain tablets.

Food groups

Anyone who is interested in eating healthily should consider planning their overall diet in relation to the five main food groups; this means taking the five groups as a starting point and working out a balanced diet by choosing the correct proportion of food each day from each of the groups. This approach still fits in with the dietary guidelines for people with diabetes (see page 13) and with those who want to eat a diet with a lower glycaemic index (see page 17). With this method there are no 'good' or 'bad' foods – just making a balanced choice.

The five main food groups required for a balanced diet

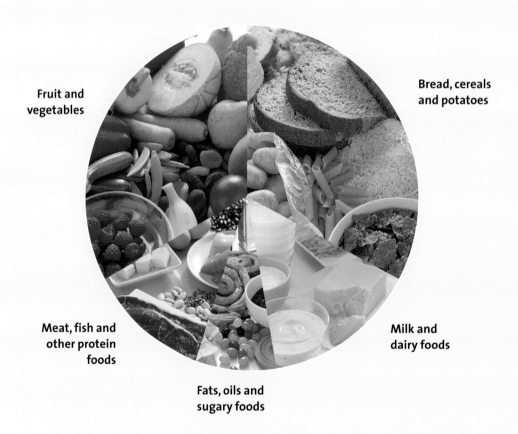

Fruit and
vegetables

Bread, cereals
and potatoes

Meat, fish and
other protein
foods

Milk and
dairy foods

Fats, oils and
sugary foods

The chart shows you the correct proportions of foods you should be eating from the different food groups – not necessarily at every meal but in your overall diet. Try to eat meals comprising more starchy foods and fruit and vegetables than food from any of the other food groups. This applies to everyone except children. With children, such a diet may be too bulky for them to eat if it is to contain sufficient nutrients and calories needed for their growth and development.

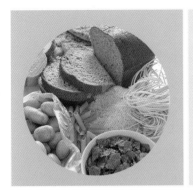

bread, cereals and potatoes

Starchy foods should form the largest portion of your diet. You should base meals and snacks around these foods when possible.

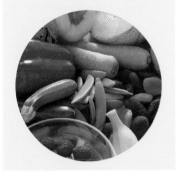

fruit and vegetables

Fruit and vegetables should make up the second largest portion. Aim to eat at least five portions every day.

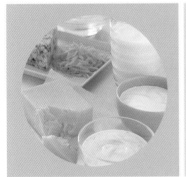

milk and dairy foods

These should make up the third largest portion of your diet. Choose low-fat dairy foods and spreads when you can.

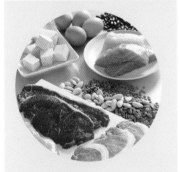

meat, fish and other protein foods

Choose lean meat and poultry, or fish, pulses or other protein foods. They should form the second smallest portion of your diet.

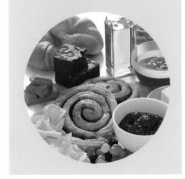

fats, oils and sugary foods

These should make up the smallest portion of your diet. Avoid fatty and sugary foods whenever possible.

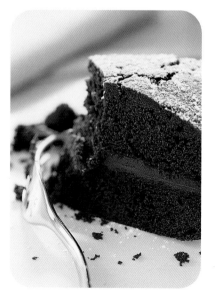

The glycaemic index

All carbohydrate foods, when digested, are reduced to glucose, but at different rates and in varying amounts depending on the specific food. The glycaemic index (GI) is a way of ranking carbohydrate foods by the effects these foods have on blood glucose levels. It is a useful way to help you to manage your carbohydrate intake and control your diabetes.

Foods are rated with a glycaemic index of between 0 and 100, based on their effect on blood glucose levels when compared with pure glucose, which scores 100 on the index as it requires no digestion and is absorbed rapidly into the blood. Foods with a high GI make blood sugar levels rise quickly soon after they are eaten, whereas foods with a lower GI release glucose into the blood much more slowly.

The idea of ranking foods this way can be a useful guide to help you understand more about choosing the right carbohydrate foods to eat for the right occasion. It can also help you to maintain good blood glucose levels more easily.

If you have diabetes, you may be taking tablets or having insulin injections, or both, but whatever your situation, a healthy diet will help to manage the condition more easily. Choosing low GI foods can help you to maintain your blood glucose levels within a reasonable range, minimizing fluctuations. There is also research that shows that people who have an overall lower glycaemic diet have healthier blood fat levels and a lower risk of heart disease into the bargain.

Starchy versus sugary foods

Carbohydrate foods are classed as either sugars or starchy foods. It used to be thought that all sugars were absorbed quickly into the bloodstream and starches were absorbed slowly. As a result, sugars and sugary foods were forbidden for people with diabetes. However, the measurement of glycaemic indices has shown that this is not the case, and that in fact some starchy foods are absorbed just as quickly as some sugary foods. A number of different factors influence the glycaemic effect of a food, including the structure of the food itself (liquids usually have a higher GI than solids, for example), and the amount of fat, protein and fibre that a food contains.

Glycaemic index values of typical foods

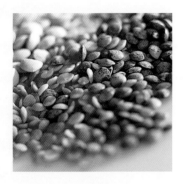

LOW

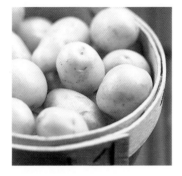

MEDIUM

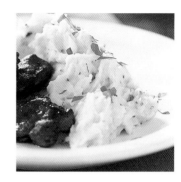

HIGH

LOW		MEDIUM		HIGH	
The following foods have a low glycaemic index:		The following foods have a medium glycaemic index:		The following foods have a high glycaemic index:	
Dried lentils, boiled	30	White basmati rice, cooked	58	White bread	70
Fettucini, cooked	32	Honey	58	Mashed potato	70
Apples, fresh	38	Ice cream, full-fat	61	Cornflakes	84
Pumpernickel bread	41	New potatoes, peeled and boiled	62	White rice, cooked	87
Porridge (made with water)	42	Wholemeal bread	69		
Green grapes	46				
Sweet potato, peeled and boiled	54				
Bananas, fresh	55				
Sweetcorn	55				

Food preparation and the glycaemic index

The way you prepare food is also significant. In general, raw food has a lower glycaemic index than cooked food. However, some canned fruits have a lower GI than the raw version, for instance peaches, apricots and pears. Mashed or puréed foods have a higher GI than foods with a more rough-cut texture as they are digested more quickly. Likewise, smaller particles of food, for example ground cereals and flour, tend to have a higher GI than non-ground foods and whole wheat.

In the past all sugary foods were forbidden for people with diabetes. GI measurements have now shown that some starchy foods are in fact absorbed just as quickly as some sugary foods.

Selecting food for its glycaemic index

Applying the glycaemic index to your food selection is not about cutting out foods with a high GI, but about balancing meals. On the whole, it may be preferable to choose low GI foods but there may be times when high GI foods are a better choice, for example in treating low blood glucose levels (see page 11). It may also be preferable to choose higher GI foods when you are ill or when you are planning to undertake high-impact physical activity.

In order to reduce the overall glycaemic index of your diet, you can incorporate more starchy carbohydrate foods with a low GI, such as bulgar wheat, pearl barley, pasta (white or wholemeal), rye bread, pumpernickel, basmati rice, sweet potato, oats, pulses and lentils. In baking, you can reduce the amount of flour and use more oat bran or rolled oats. Or you can combine foods or dishes with a lower GI, such as vegetables, fruit and pulses, with foods or dishes that have a higher GI, to reduce the overall effect on blood glucose levels.

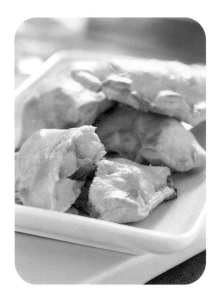

Applying the glycaemic index to your food selection is not about cutting out foods with a high glycaemic index, but about balancing meals.

Recommended dietary changes for someone with diabetes

	Sample day's eating	Recommended food if you have diabetes
Breakfast	Toast	Have porridge oats or a bran cereal AND add fruit and low-fat milk
Morning snack	Biscuits	Replace with fresh fruit
Lunch	Wholemeal bread sandwich	Use pumpernickel bread or a multigrain bread
Afternoon snack	Crisps	Replace with fresh fruit
Evening meal	Chicken casserole with potatoes	Add lentils, cooked beans or pearl barley. Serve with pasta or noodles

A balancing act

It is important to remember that the glycaemic index is measured for individual foods, but we tend to eat combinations of foods. Combining foods with a lower GI (fruit, vegetables and pulses) with foods that have a higher GI helps you to achieve easier blood glucose control. Low GI foods can also help you to control your appetite by making you feel fuller for longer – with the result that you eat less.

It is important not to worry about every single meal that you eat. Try to eat lower GI foods on a regular basis if you can, but don't lose sleep over it. Remember it's not about cutting out high GI foods altogether. Some combinations of foods are just meant for each other – in terms of both taste and nutrition – whatever the glycaemic effects when combined. You may find that simply eating more fruit and vegetables makes a difference to your blood glucose control and your general health and wellbeing.

The recipes in this book have all been given a GI rating – low (below 55), medium (55–70) or high (over 70) – for your convenience, but you can apply the concept of glycaemic indices to your meal planning in a number of ways:

❶ Combine foods of a lower glycaemic index (fruit, vegetables and pulses) with foods with a higher GI

❷ Choose carbohydrate foods with a low GI as the accompaniment to your meal, for example pasta rather than potatoes with meat, fish and vegetables

❸ Select a different low GI food to eat at each meal, for example eat oats at breakfast, rye bread at lunch and pasta or pulses at supper time

Food checklist

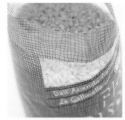

Choose wholegrain varieties of pasta, rice, bread and cereals as they are higher in fibre

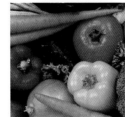

Eat lots of fruit and vegetables – fresh, frozen, dried or canned (five portions a day)

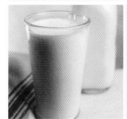

Use lower-fat dairy products to reduce animal fat or saturated fat intake

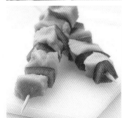

Choose lean cuts of meat, and always remove skin from poultry

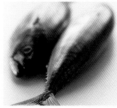

Eat more fish

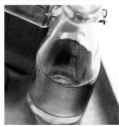

Use foods high in monounsaturated and polyunsaturated fat, and cut down on saturated fat

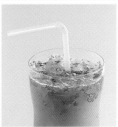

Avoid sugary drinks

Sample menus

Menu planning requires forward thinking, which can be a challenge, when, as well as juggling everything that life throws at you, you also have to manage your diabetes. One thing you can do to make life easier is to plan ahead, shop in advance and have all the ingredients that you need at hand ready to make speedy meals.

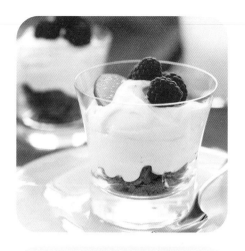

midweek vegetarian supper

herbed pasta with roasted cherry tomatoes (see page 32)

griddled pineapple and ginger (see page 108)

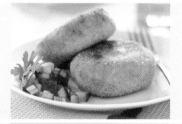

vegetarian lunch

herby bean cakes (see page 56)

tropical fruit salad (see page 110)

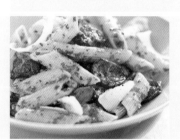

entertaining with style and speed

fresh figs with ricotta cheese and Parma ham
   (see page 104)

chicken tagine with fruity couscous (see page 42)

baked red fruits with crispy topping (see page 107)

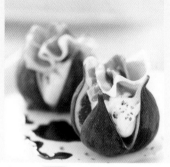

friends for dinner

prawn and noodle soup (see page 46)

thai chicken curry with citrus rice (see page 35)

grilled nectarines with mint vanilla cream
   (see page 114)

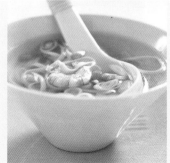

one-pot supper

hearty seafood soup (see page 83)

irish soda bread (see page 138)

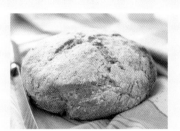

romantic supper

minted lamb with potato rosti (see page 90)

individual lime and raspberry cheesecakes (see page 112)

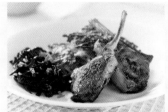

elegant supper

teriyaki salmon on noodles (see page 48)

watermelon granita (see page 111)

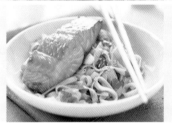

brunch dishes

all-day breakfast (see page 74)

smoked haddock and poached egg muffins (see page 133)

tasty open toasties (see page 126)

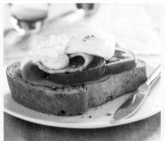

children's favourites

mozzarella burgers (see page 129)

spring onion and potato pasties (see page 76)

super smoothies (see page 116)

pitta with citrus chicken brochettes (see page 122)

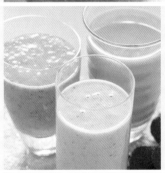

low-calorie dishes

thai beef and noodle salad (see page 50)

mixed mushroom risotto (see page 38)

pearl barley salad with griddled chicken (see page 44)

nutty citrus wild rice salad (page 34)

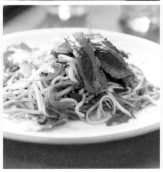

living with diabetes

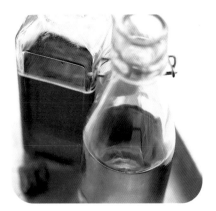

If you have diabetes, you will inevitably have to make some changes to your way of life. However, simply by giving more careful consideration to your diet in terms of food choice, food shopping, cooking and eating, you should be able to continue with your normal activities. Having diabetes does not mean going without life's pleasures; it just means adhering to the principles of a healthy diet that everyone should already be following and monitoring your condition with the help of healthcare professionals.

Healthy cooking

Try to incorporate the dietary guidelines on page 13, and balance the proportions of different foods in your diet (see page 14). You can easily adapt favourite recipes to be lower in fat (see below) and salt, and balance simple meals by serving them with extra foods such as bread, salad or vegetables.

Reducing your fat intake

There are a number of ways you can cut down on fat in cooking:

- Grill, bake, poach, steam, dry roast or dry fry foods rather than fry them in oil

- Use a low-fat spread or low-fat cheese spread in place of full-fat butter or margarine

- Make a paste with flour and liquid to thicken sauces, rather than using flour and butter to make a traditional roux-based sauce

- Use lean cuts of meat and poultry and remove visible fat and skin before cooking

- Skim off fat after cooking

- Eat more meat alternatives such as pulses, quorn, tofu and soya-textured-protein products

- Use more starchy carbohydrate foods such as bulgar wheat, pasta, rice and other cereals as a basis for main meals

Get into the habit of using the right sort of fat

1. Use oils and spreads that are high in monounsaturated fats (olive oil, rapeseed oil and nut oils) or polyunsaturated fats (sunflower, safflower, soya, corn or grapeseed oils)

2. Look out for unsalted versions of spreads and fats to reduce your sodium intake

Top 10 shopping tips

❶ Choose low-fat dairy products, such as skimmed or semi-skimmed milk, low-fat yogurts and low- or reduced-fat spreads instead of butter. Use light crème fraîche or fromage frais in place of cream

❷ Buy lean meat and poultry

❸ Buy canned fish to keep in your storecupboard

❹ Stock up with a range of cooking oils, such as sesame, walnut and olive, and a good range of spices and dried, bottled or frozen herbs

❺ Mustard, flavoured vinegars, balsamic vinegar, soy sauce, Thai fish sauce, Worcestershire sauce and Tabasco are also useful storecupboard items

❻ Look out for alternative seasonings such as seaweed salt and sea salt. Although these products still contain as much sodium, you use less. Also look for reduced-sodium stock cubes

❼ Use fat-free or low-calorie dressings for quick and easy flavourings, but watch the sodium content

❽ Cereals like porridge oats, rice, pasta, pearl barley, bulgar wheat and dried beans and pulses can form the basis of a hearty meal

❾ Canned tomatoes and sweetcorn supplement the vegetables in a meal

❿ Canned fruits and dried fruits are also useful reserves

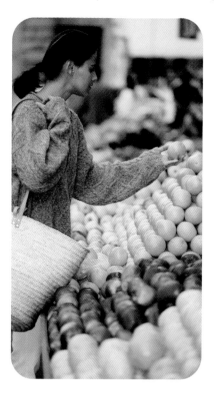

Healthy eating is easily achievable. All it means is that you must give more careful consideration to your diet, food shopping, cooking and lifestyle.

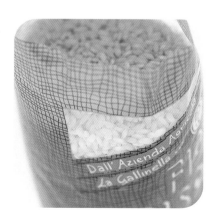

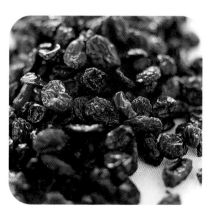

Understanding food labels

Food labels provide information about the nutritional content of food. When comparing food labels, you need to consider how the food will fit into your overall diet – how much of it you are likely to eat and how often, and whether it is a good choice in terms of calorie, fat and carbohydrate content. You may feel that certain foods are high in fat and calories, and therefore not a good choice on an everyday basis, but those foods you can save for occasional treats. The example below shows how to read a food label and get the information you need.

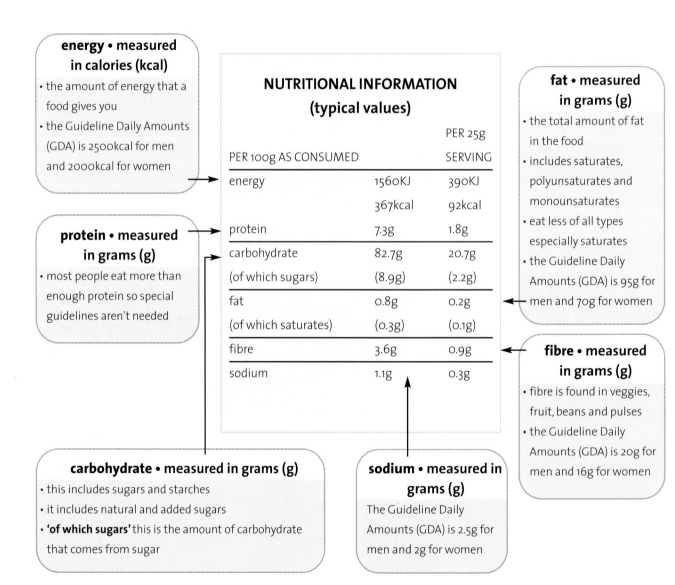

energy • measured in calories (kcal)
- the amount of energy that a food gives you
- the Guideline Daily Amounts (GDA) is 2500kcal for men and 2000kcal for women

protein • measured in grams (g)
- most people eat more than enough protein so special guidelines aren't needed

carbohydrate • measured in grams (g)
- this includes sugars and starches
- it includes natural and added sugars
- **'of which sugars'** this is the amount of carbohydrate that comes from sugar

NUTRITIONAL INFORMATION (typical values)

PER 100g AS CONSUMED		PER 25g SERVING
energy	1560KJ	390KJ
	367kcal	92kcal
protein	7.3g	1.8g
carbohydrate	82.7g	20.7g
(of which sugars)	(8.9g)	(2.2g)
fat	0.8g	0.2g
(of which saturates)	(0.3g)	(0.1g)
fibre	3.6g	0.9g
sodium	1.1g	0.3g

fat • measured in grams (g)
- the total amount of fat in the food
- includes saturates, polyunsaturates and monounsaturates
- eat less of all types especially saturates
- the Guideline Daily Amounts (GDA) is 95g for men and 70g for women

fibre • measured in grams (g)
- fibre is found in veggies, fruit, beans and pulses
- the Guideline Daily Amounts (GDA) is 20g for men and 16g for women

sodium • measured in grams (g)
The Guideline Daily Amounts (GDA) is 2.5g for men and 2g for women

Eating out

Having diabetes does not mean that you can't enjoy meals out with friends and family. It does, however, mean that you need to take more care with meal planning and monitoring your diabetes. You may need to seek advice from your doctor or diabetes nurse if you are going to be eating at an unusual time of day and your medication needs adjustment. If your diabetes is treated with diet alone, or a combination of diet and tablets, the timing will not be so crucial. If you have insulin injections, however, you need to ensure that your meal will not be delayed.

Simple self-help measures

Simple measures, such as having a small snack like a banana before you go out, or delaying your injection until you arrive at the restaurant or party, may be all that is needed. You can always ask for some bread to nibble if you are a little behind your normal schedule. Never drink alcohol on an empty stomach because alcohol lowers your blood glucose level and you therefore risk hypoglycaemia (see page 11). As a general rule, drink alcohol with food rather than before a meal or before food is served.

If you eat out only rarely, you should be able to enjoy a special occasion and not worry too much about the additional calories or fat – as long as your blood glucose level is under control.

Eating out regularly

If you eat out regularly, then you need to choose your food more carefully. Try to stick to one or two courses rather than a full menu all the time, and avoid high-fat foods such as pies, creamy sauces and soups, fried foods and chips. Make sure you have plenty of vegetables, salad and carbohydrate-based dishes. Pasta or rice with pulses, tomato- and vegetable-based sauces are very good choices. Avoid eating heavy puddings laden with cream on a regular basis.

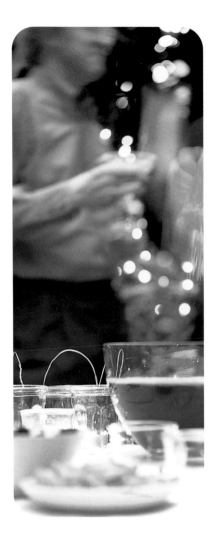

Having diabetes does not mean that you cannot enjoy special celebrations or the occasional meal out.

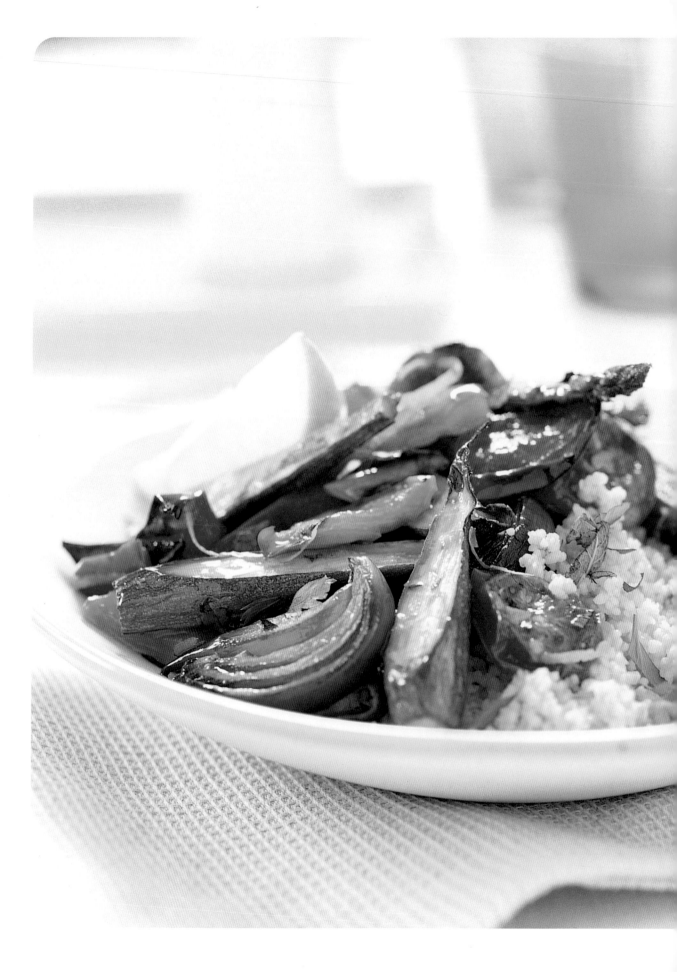

rice, pasta and other grains

You can create complete meals in no time at all by using different combinations of vegetables, meat and fish with starchy carbohydrate foods such as rice, pasta and grains.

Since they have a lower glycaemic index, try including pasta and rice in your meals instead of potatoes. You can add ready-made sauces to rice and pasta for meals in a flash. Choose tomato- or vegetable-based sauces rather than creamy ones with lots of cheese.

Pasta is made from hard-wheat semolina with a high protein content which gives it a low glycaemic index. Different sorts of pasta have different glycaemic indices – usually thicker shapes have a lower index than thinner ones. Try other grains, too, such as bulgar wheat and pearl barley, and look out for quick-cooking versions to cut down on cooking times.

Similarly to pasta the glycaemic index of rice varies: due to the type of starch it contains, basmati rice has a lower glycaemic index than other types of long-grain rice. Add pulses or beans to the rice to reduce the glycaemic load.

pasta with prawns, peas and mint

375 g (12 oz) dried pasta shapes

200 g (7 oz) frozen peas

1 tablespoon olive oil

1 onion, sliced

1 garlic clove, crushed

150 ml (¼ pint) dry white wine

200 g (7 oz) cooked tiger prawns

6 tablespoons light crème fraîche

2 tablespoons freshly grated
   Parmesan cheese

2 tablespoons chopped mint

salt and pepper

mint leaves, to garnish

1 Cook the pasta according to packet instructions, add the peas 2 minutes before the end of cooking time. Drain.

2 Meanwhile heat the oil in a nonstick saucepan, add the onion and garlic and fry for 2–3 minutes until they begin to soften.

3 Add the wine to the pan, bring to the boil and reduce by about a half.

4 Stir in the prawns, crème fraîche, Parmesan and mint and heat through. Season to taste with salt and pepper. Toss the sauce through the pasta and serve garnished with mint leaves.

NUTRITIONAL FACTS

GI rating: LOW

- Kcals – 444
- Protein – 25 g
- Carbohydrate – 75 g
- Fat – 11 g

NUTRITIONAL TIP

Shellfish are a source of cholesterol; however they can be included in your diet as blood cholesterol is more affected by the amount of saturated fat in a diet and other factors such as weight.

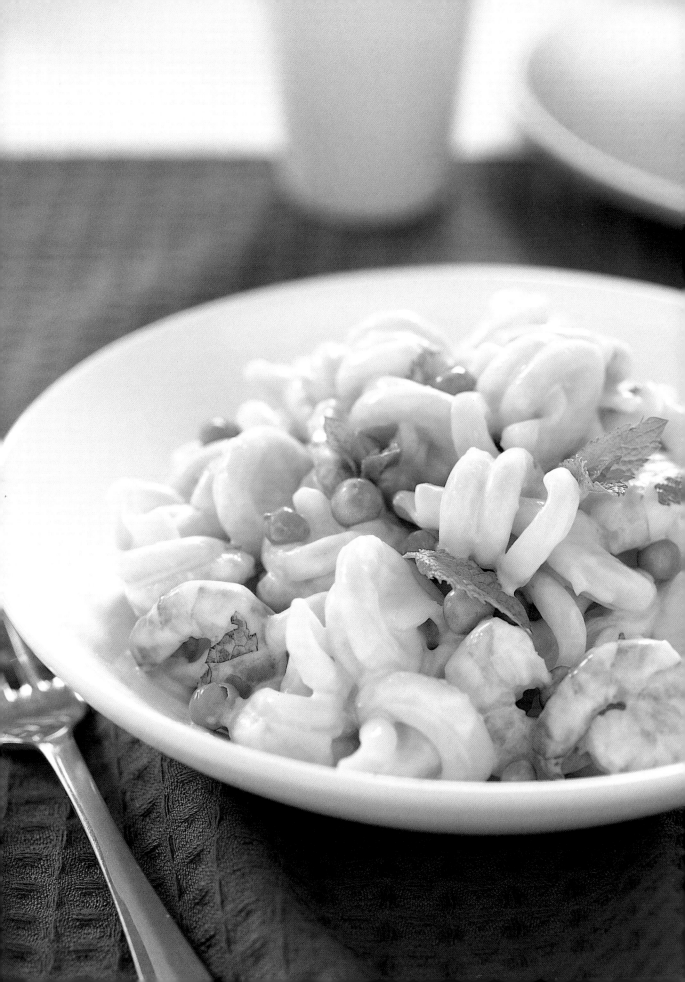

pork balls with tomato sauce and spaghetti

375 g (12 oz) dried spaghetti

300 g (10 oz) minced pork

1 onion, finely chopped

1 garlic clove, crushed

½ teaspoon paprika

2 teaspoons tomato purée

700 g (1 lb 6 oz) jar passata

salt and pepper

1 Cook the spaghetti according to packet instructions.

2 Meanwhile, mix together the mince, onion, garlic and paprika and season with salt and pepper. Shape the mixture into 12 balls.

3 Place the meatballs on a grill pan and cook under a preheated grill for 6–7 minutes, turning occasionally, until browned and cooked through.

4 Drain the spaghetti, return it to the saucepan and stir in the tomato purée, passata and the meatballs. Season to taste with salt and pepper, heat through and serve.

NUTRITIONAL FACTS

GI rating: LOW

- Kcals – 486
- Protein – 27 g
- Carbohydrate – 78 g
- Fat – 9 g

NUTRITIONAL TIP

Dry roast meatballs rather than frying them so that you reduce your intake of fat.

pasta with tomato, spinach and ricotta sauce

375 g (12 oz) dried pasta shapes

1 teaspoon olive oil

1 garlic clove, crushed

1 onion, sliced

½ teaspoon dried chilli flakes

700 g (1 lb 6 oz) jar passata

225 g (7½ oz) baby spinach leaves

150 g (5 oz) ricotta cheese

salt and pepper

1 Cook the pasta according to packet instructions and drain.

2 Meanwhile, heat the oil in a saucepan, add the garlic and onion and fry for 3–4 minutes. Add the chilli flakes and continue to fry for 1 minute.

3 Stir in the passata and simmer for 2 minutes. Add the spinach and ricotta, stir until the spinach has wilted then simmer for 3–4 minutes.

4 Toss the pasta through the sauce, season to taste with salt and pepper and serve.

NUTRITIONAL FACTS

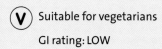 Suitable for vegetarians

GI rating: LOW

- Kcals – 432
- Protein – 18 g
- Carbohydrate – 79 g
- Fat – 7 g

NUTRITIONAL TIP

Ricotta is a soft cheese which can be used in sauces. It has a low to medium fat content.

herbed pasta with roasted cherry tomatoes

375 g (12 oz) dried pasta shapes

200 g (7 oz) cherry tomatoes, halved

2 tablespoons pesto

1 tablespoon white wine vinegar

2 tablespoons capers, drained

2 anchovy fillets, chopped (optional)

2 tablespoons chopped mixed herbs
  (such as parsley and basil)

salt and pepper

Parmesan cheese shavings, to garnish

crisp green salad, to serve

1 Cook the pasta according to packet instructions and drain.

2 Meanwhile, place the tomatoes under a preheated hot grill and cook for about 15 minutes until slightly charred and beginning to dry out.

3 Place the pesto, vinegar, capers, anchovies and herbs in a food processor or blender and blend until almost smooth but retaining a little texture.

4 Toss the sauce through the hot pasta with the tomatoes, season to taste with salt and pepper and serve with some Parmesan shavings and a crisp green salad.

NUTRITIONAL FACTS

(V) Suitable for vegetarians

GI rating: LOW

- Kcals – 406
- Protein – 15 g
- Carbohydrate – 72 g
- Fat – 7 g

NUTRITIONAL TIP

Pasta is a good staple for use in vegetarian meals as it is also a source of protein.

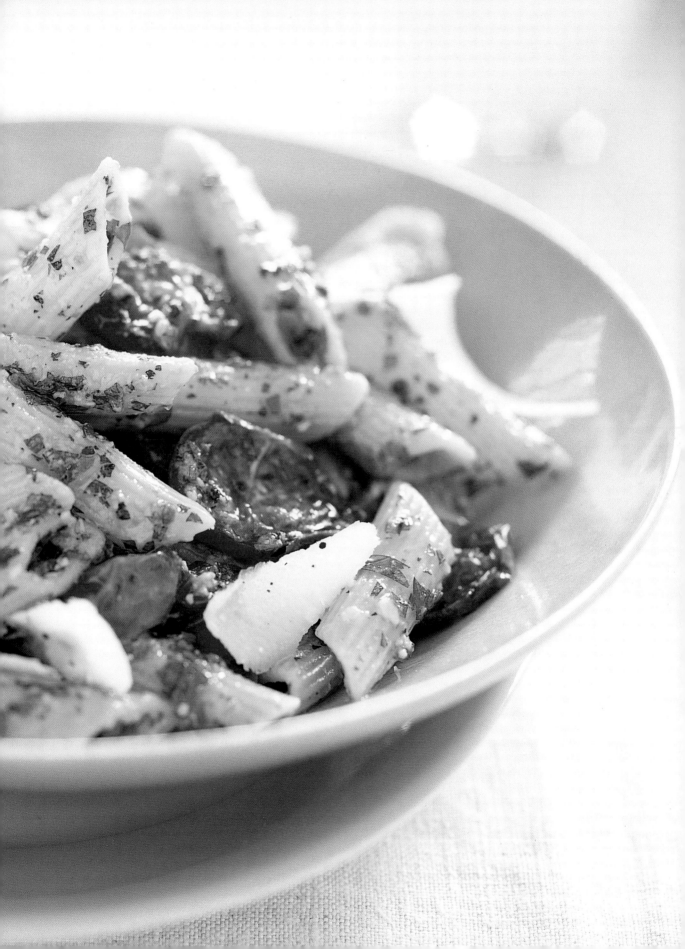

nutty citrus wild rice salad

200 g (7 oz) mixed long grain and
  wild rice

1 tablespoon wholegrain mustard

grated rind and juice of 1 large orange

1 orange, segmented

4 spring onions, sliced

12 cherry tomatoes, quartered

75 g (3 oz) mixed seeds (such as
  pumpkin, sunflower and pinenuts),
  toasted

50 g (2 oz) feta cheese, crumbled

60 g (2½ oz) watercress, chopped

2 tablespoons chopped parsley

salt and pepper

1 Cook the rice according to packet instructions. Drain, then refresh under cold running water.

2 Mix together the mustard, and the orange rind and juice. Stir through the rice then add the orange segments, spring onions, tomatoes, mixed seeds, feta, watercress and parsley. Season to taste with salt and pepper and serve.

NUTRITIONAL FACTS

 Suitable for vegetarians

GI rating: LOW

- Kcals – 316
- Protein – 10 g
- Carbohydrate – 50 g
- Fat – 9 g

NUTRITIONAL TIP

Feta cheese has a high water content and a high sodium content. It is very good in salads, but should be used sparingly.

thai chicken curry with citrus rice

1 Heat the oil in a pan and add the lemon grass, lime leaves, chilli, ginger, onion and garlic, and fry for 2 minutes.

2 Add the peppers and chicken and continue to fry for 5 minutes.

3 Pour in the coconut milk and the stock and simmer for a further 10 minutes or until the chicken is cooked through.

4 Stir in half of the coriander and season to taste with salt and pepper.

5 Meanwhile, put the rice into a pan of lightly salted boiling water with half the lime rind and juice. Cook according to packet instructions until tender, then drain. Stir in the remaining lime rind and juice and coriander. Serve with the curry.

1 tablespoon sunflower oil

1 lemon grass stalk, cut into 4

2 kaffir lime leaves, halved

1–2 red chillies, finely chopped

2.5 cm (1 inch) piece fresh root ginger, peeled and grated

1 onion, finely chopped

1 garlic clove, crushed

1 red pepper, cored, deseeded and chopped

1 green pepper, cored, deseeded and chopped

3 boneless, skinless chicken breasts, chopped

400 g (13 oz) can reduced fat coconut milk

150 ml (¼ pint) chicken stock

4 tablespoons chopped coriander leaves

250 g (8 oz) basmati rice

grated rind and juice of 2 limes

salt and pepper

NUTRITIONAL FACTS

GI rating: MEDIUM

- Kcals – 451
- Protein – 38 g
- Carbohydrate – 61 g
- Fat – 6 g

NUTRITIONAL TIP

Coconut milk is high in saturated fat and calories, so look out for the reduced fat version and use sparingly.

smoked salmon and cream cheese risotto

2 teaspoons olive oil

1 onion, finely chopped

2 garlic cloves, crushed

300 g (10 oz) risotto rice

150 ml (¼ pint) dry white wine

900 ml (1½ pints) simmering
  vegetable stock

125 g (4 oz) light cream cheese

125 g (4 oz) smoked salmon, chopped

4 tablespoons chopped herbs (such as
  chives, parsley or dill)

salt and pepper

1 Heat the oil in a large saucepan, add the onion and garlic and fry for 2–3 minutes until they begin to soften.

2 Stir in the rice and continue to cook for 1 minute. Add the wine and cook, stirring, until the wine has been absorbed.

3 Reduce the heat and add the stock a little at a time, stirring continuously, and allowing each amount of stock to be absorbed before adding the next. Continue until all the stock has been absorbed.

4 Stir in the cream cheese, smoked salmon and herbs, season to taste with salt and pepper and serve.

NUTRITIONAL FACTS

GI rating: MEDIUM

- Kcals – 428
- Protein – 17 g
- Carbohydrate – 60 g
- Fat – 8 g

NUTRITIONAL TIP

Smoked salmon is an oily fish which contains omega-3 fatty acids, which helps to protect against heart disease. Try to eat oily fish at least once a week.

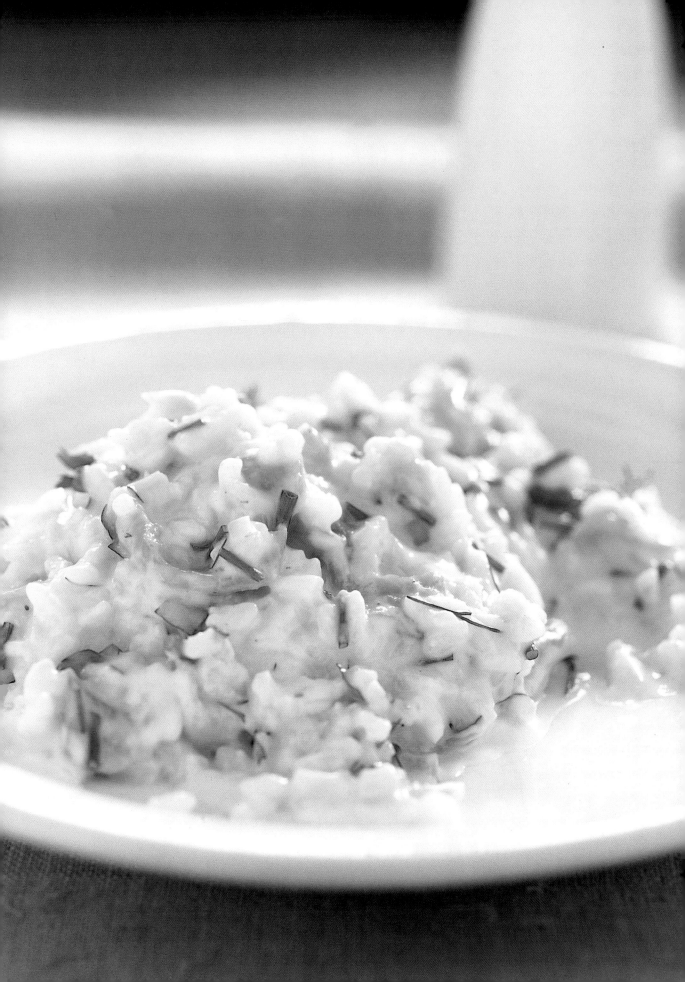

mixed mushroom risotto

1 Place the dried mushrooms in a bowl, cover with a cup of boiling water and set aside.

2 Heat a little of the oil in a large frying pan, add the onion and garlic and fry for 2–3 minutes until beginning to soften.

3 Add the rice and continue to cook for 1 minute, stirring to coat the rice in the oil. Add the wine and cook, stirring, until it has been absorbed.

4 Reduce the heat and add the stock a little at a time, stirring continuously. Allow each amount of stock to be absorbed before adding the next. Continue until all the stock has been absorbed, then add the porcini mushrooms and their liquid.

5 Heat the remaining oil in another saucepan and fry the fresh mushrooms until cooked. Stir into the rice mixture with the parsley and Parmesan, season to taste with salt and pepper and serve.

25 g (1 oz) dried porcini mushrooms
1 tablespoon olive oil
1 onion, finely chopped
2 garlic cloves, crushed
300 g (10 oz) risotto rice
150 ml (¼ pint) dry white wine
900 ml (1½ pints) simmering
   vegetable stock
500 g (1 lb) mixed mushrooms (such as
   flat cap, button and brown)
handful of chopped parsley
25 g (1 oz) Parmesan cheese, grated
salt and pepper

NUTRITIONAL FACTS

 Suitable for vegetarians
GI rating: MEDIUM

- Kcals – 407
- Protein – 13 g
- Carbohydrate – 60 g
- Fat – 9 g

NUTRITIONAL TIP

Parmesan cheese is a hard cheese; it is high in fat so grate finely and use sparingly.

vegetable biryani

1 Cook the rice in boiling water according to packet instructions. Drain.

2 Meanwhile, heat the oil in a nonstick saucepan, add the carrots, potato, ginger and garlic and fry for 10 minutes until beginning to soften.

3 Stir in the cauliflower, beans, curry paste, turmeric and cinnamon and cook for 1 minute.

4 Stir in the yogurt and raisins. Pile the rice on to the vegetable mixture. Cover and cook over a low heat for 10 minutes, checking from time to time that it isn't sticking to the pan.

5 Turn the biryani into a large serving dish, sprinkle with the nuts and coriander and serve.

250 g (8 oz) long-grain rice

1 tablespoon olive oil

2 carrots, chopped

1 large potato, chopped

1 tablespoon grated fresh root ginger

2 garlic cloves, crushed

150 g (5 oz) cauliflower florets

100 g (3½ oz) green beans, halved

1 tablespoon hot curry paste

1 teaspoon turmeric

½ teaspoon ground cinnamon

150 g (5 oz) plain yogurt

25 g (1 oz) raisins

50 g (2 oz) cashew nuts, toasted

2 tablespoons chopped coriander
    leaves

NUTRITIONAL FACTS

 Suitable for vegetarians

GI rating: MEDIUM

- Kcals – 450
- Protein – 12 g
- Carbohydrate – 72 g
- Fat – 11 g

NUTRITIONAL TIP

Nuts are high in fat but they are also a good source of protein and fibre in the diet.

couscous with grilled vegetables

300 g (10 oz) couscous

500 ml (17 fl oz) boiling water

2 red peppers, cored, deseeded
and quartered

1 orange pepper, cored, deseeded
and quartered

6 baby courgettes, halved lengthways

2 red onions, cut into wedges

24 cherry tomatoes

2 garlic cloves, finely sliced

2 tablespoons olive oil

100 g (3½ oz) asparagus spears

grated rind and juice of 1 lemon

4 tablespoons chopped herbs (such as
parsley or mint)

salt and pepper

1 Tip the couscous into a large bowl, pour over the water, cover and set aside for 10 minutes while preparing the remaining ingredients.

2 Place the peppers, courgettes, onions, tomatoes and garlic in a grill pan in one layer, drizzle over the oil and cook under a preheated hot grill for 5–6 minutes, turning the vegetables occasionally.

3 Add the asparagus to the pan and continue to grill for 2–3 minutes until the vegetables are tender and lightly charred. When they are cool enough to handle, remove the skins from the peppers and discard.

4 Fork through the couscous to separate the grains. Toss with the vegetables, lime rind and juice, and herbs, season to taste with salt and pepper and serve.

NUTRITIONAL FACTS

 Suitable for vegetarians

GI rating: MEDIUM

O Kcals – 470

O Protein – 12 g

O Carbohydrate – 85 g

O Fat – 8 g

NUTRITIONAL TIP

Cherry tomatoes are a good source of antioxidants in the diet. Antioxidants help to improve general health and are thought to slow down the ageing process in the body.

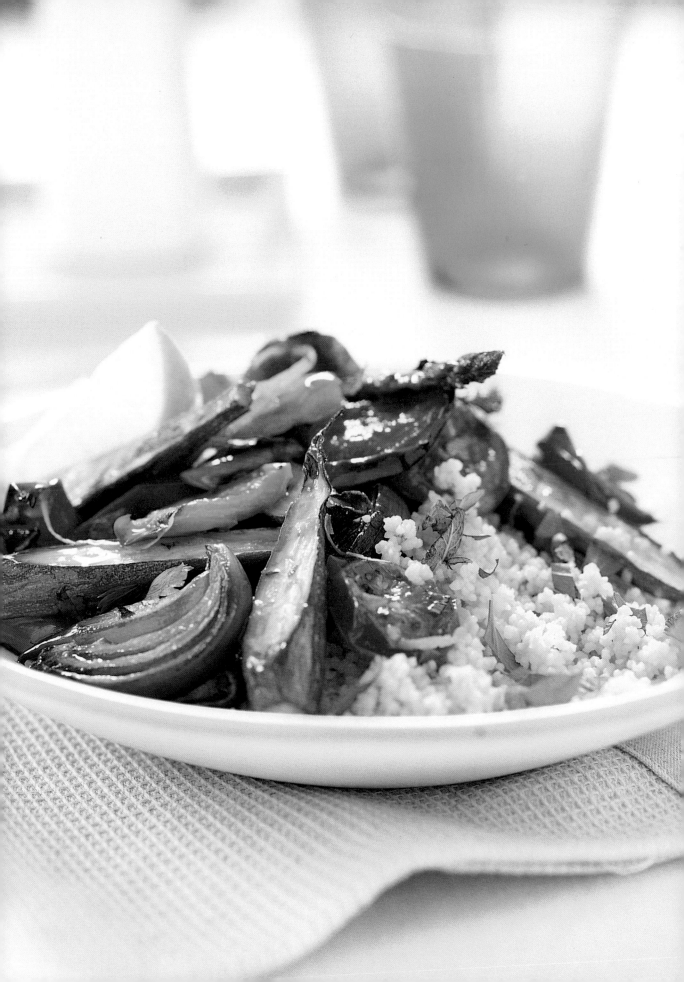

chicken tagine with fruity couscous

1 Heat the oil in a large casserole. Add the chicken, onion and garlic and fry gently for 3–4 minutes until the chicken is beginning to brown.

2 Stir in the cumin, ginger and paprika and fry for 1 minute. Add the apricots, chickpeas, saffron, stock, lemon rind and juice, and olives to the pan, cover and simmer for 15 minutes.

3 Meanwhile, place the couscous in a bowl with the sultanas and pour over the boiling water. Leave to soak for about 5 minutes until the water has been absorbed, fluffing up the grains from time to time with a fork.

4 Stir the mint into the couscous and the parsley into the chicken tagine. Season to taste with salt and pepper. Serve the tagine on top of the couscous with plenty of the cooking liquid.

1 tablespoon olive oil

8 medium boneless, skinless
   chicken thighs

1 large onion, chopped

2 garlic cloves, crushed

1 teaspoon ground cumin

½ teaspoon ground ginger

1 teaspoon paprika

100 g (3½ oz) ready-to-eat dried
   apricots, halved

400 g (13 oz) can chickpeas, drained
   and rinsed

¼ teaspoon saffron threads

450 ml (¾ pint) chicken stock

grated rind and juice of ½ lemon

100 g (3½ oz) pitted green olives

300 g (10 oz) couscous

100 g (3½ oz) sultanas

500 ml (17 fl oz) boiling water

4 tablespoons chopped mint

4 tablespoons chopped flat leaf parsley

salt and pepper

NUTRITIONAL FACTS

GI rating: MEDIUM

- Kcals – 544
- Protein – 35 g
- Carbohydrate – 67 g
- Fat – 15 g

NUTRITIONAL TIP

This recipe can be served as a vegetarian dish without the chicken; it is just as nutritious and delicious.

roasted tomato and bulgar wheat salad

250 g (8 oz) bulgar wheat

300 g (10 oz) cherry tomatoes, halved

2 red peppers, cored, deseeded and
   quartered

2 tablespoons olive oil

25 g (1 oz) pine nuts, toasted

400 g (13 oz) can artichoke hearts,
   drained

50 g (2 oz) feta cheese, crumbled

2 tablespoons chopped parsley

grated rind and juice of 1 lemon

1 tablespoon clear honey

2 teaspoons Dijon mustard

salt and pepper

1 Place the bulgar wheat in a large bowl, cover with boiling water and leave to soak for 10–15 minutes until the grains are tender. Drain well.

2 Meanwhile, place the tomatoes and peppers on a grill pan, drizzle with half the oil and season with salt and pepper. Place under a preheated hot grill for 5–7 minutes, turning occasionally, until charred and tender.

3 Remove and discard the skin from the peppers, slice the flesh and add to the bulgar wheat, along with the tomatoes, pine nuts, artichoke hearts, feta and parsley.

4 Whisk together the lemon rind and juice, honey, mustard and the remaining oil, and drizzle over the salad. Season to taste with salt and pepper, toss to combine and serve.

NUTRITIONAL FACTS

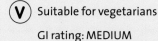 Suitable for vegetarians

    GI rating: MEDIUM

- Kcals – 380
- Protein – 11 g
- Carbohydrate – 60 g
- Fat – 11 g

NUTRITIONAL TIP

Artichokes are good sources of folate and potassium in the diet. Tinned artichokes can be as nutritious as fresh ones.

pearl barley salad with griddled chicken

1 Brush each chicken piece with a little oil. Heat a griddle until hot and cook the chicken for 4–5 minutes on each side until cooked and browned. Cut each breast into 4 slices.

2 Stir the remaining oil into the barley, and add the onion, chilli, coriander, lime rind and juice, and red pepper. Season to taste with salt and pepper and stir to combine.

3 Serve the barley topped with the chicken, garnished with parsley and lime wedges.

4 boneless, skinless chicken breasts

1 tablespoon olive oil

125 g (4 oz) pearl barley, cooked to packet instructions

1 red onion, finely chopped

1 red chilli, finely chopped

4 tablespoons chopped coriander leaves

grated rind and juice of 2 limes

1 red pepper, cored, deseeded and finely chopped

salt and pepper

TO GARNISH

parsley sprigs

lime wedges

NUTRITIONAL FACTS

GI rating: LOW

- Kcals – 274
- Protein – 27 g
- Carbohydrate – 31 g
- Fat – 5 g

NUTRITIONAL TIP

Pearl barley is high in soluble fibre and can be used as a substitute for rice.

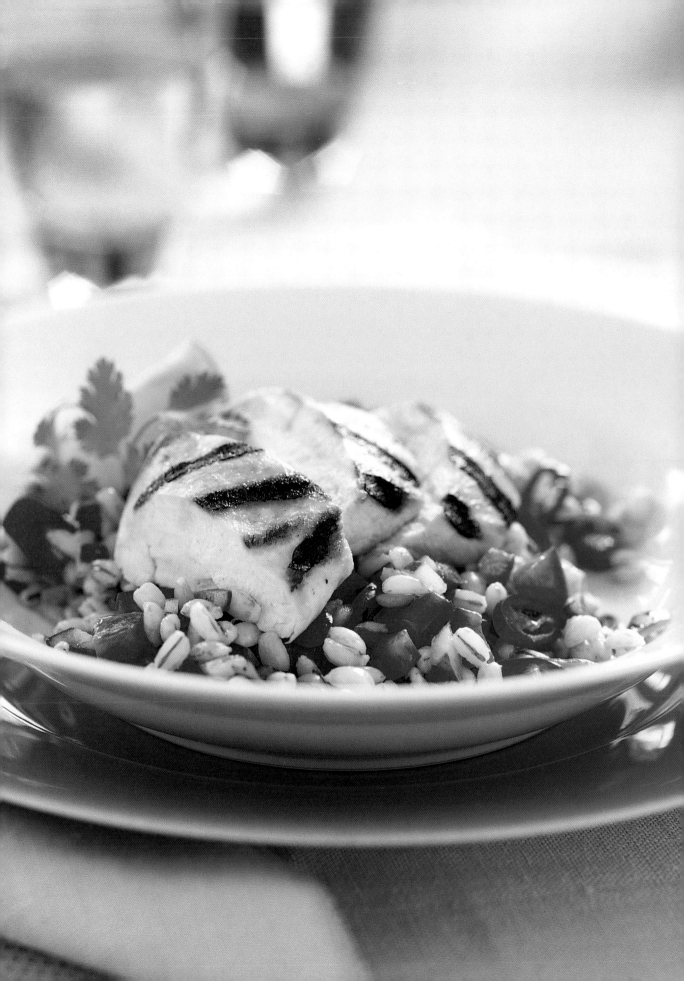

prawn and noodle soup

900 ml (1½ pints) vegetable or
  chicken stock
2 kaffir lime leaves
1 lemon grass stalk, lightly bruised
150 g (5 oz) dried egg noodles
50 g (2 oz) frozen peas
50 g (2 oz) frozen sweetcorn
100 g (3½ oz) large, cooked and peeled
  prawns
4 spring onions, sliced
2 teaspoons soy sauce

1 Put the stock into a saucepan with the lime leaves and lemon grass, bring to the boil and simmer for 10 minutes.

2 Add the noodles to the stock and cook according to packet instructions. After 2 minutes, add the peas, sweetcorn, prawns, spring onions and soy sauce. Serve in individual bowls.

NUTRITIONAL FACTS

GI rating: LOW

- Kcals – 187
- Protein – 10 g
- Carbohydrate – 30 g
- Fat – 3 g

NUTRITIONAL TIP

Frozen vegetables can be just as nutritious as fresh vegetables. As well as keeping a good colour and flavour most of the nutrients are retained.

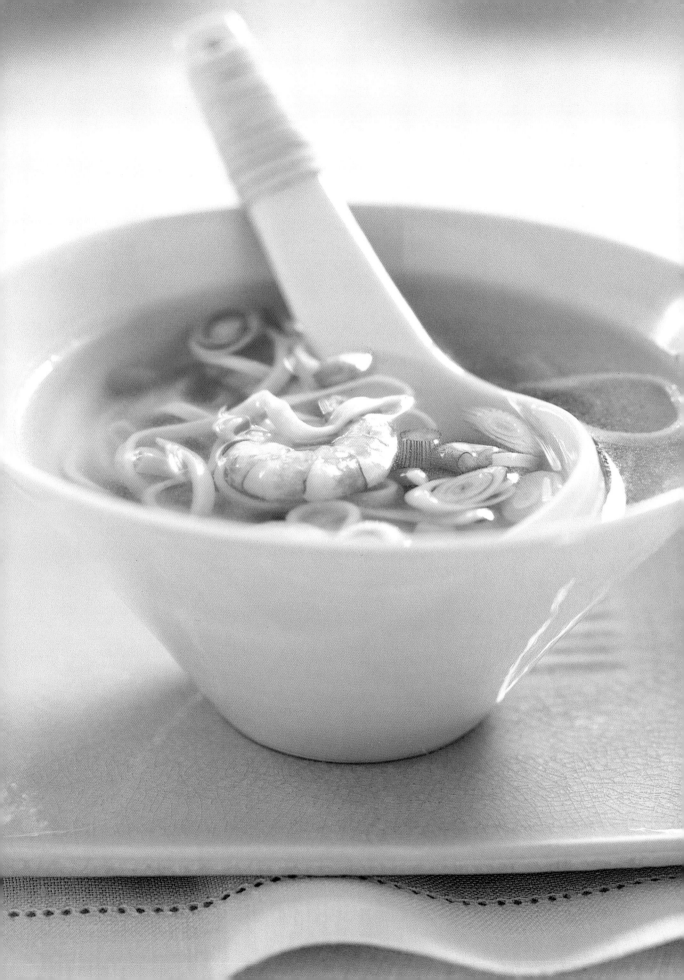

teriyaki salmon on noodles

1 Place the salmon on a foil-lined grill pan. Mix together the soy sauce, sherry, sugar, garlic, ginger, half of the oil and the water. Brush half of the marinade over the salmon and set aside for 10 minutes.

2 Cook the salmon under a preheated hot grill for 5–6 minutes, turning it halfway through the cooking time and brushing with a little more of the marinade.

3 Meanwhile, heat the remaining oil in a saucepan, add the sesame seeds and spring onions and fry for 1 minute.

4 Add the noodles and any remaining marinade to the saucepan and heat through. Stir in the coriander. Serve the salmon on a bed of noodles.

4 pieces skinless salmon fillet, about 125 g (4 oz) each
2 tablespoons soy sauce
1 tablespoon dry sherry
2 tablespoons soft brown sugar
2 garlic cloves, crushed
1 teaspoon grated fresh root ginger
1 tablespoon sesame oil
2 tablespoons water
2 tablespoons sesame seeds
2 spring onions, chopped
250 g (8 oz) dried rice noodles, cooked according to packet instructions
3 tablespoons chopped coriander leaves

NUTRITIONAL FACTS

(V) Suitable for vegetarians
GI rating: LOW

- Kcals – 504
- Protein – 30 g
- Carbohydrate – 50 g
- Fat – 20 g

NUTRITIONAL TIP
Sesame seeds are a source of calcium and magnesium and an excellent addition to exotic dishes.

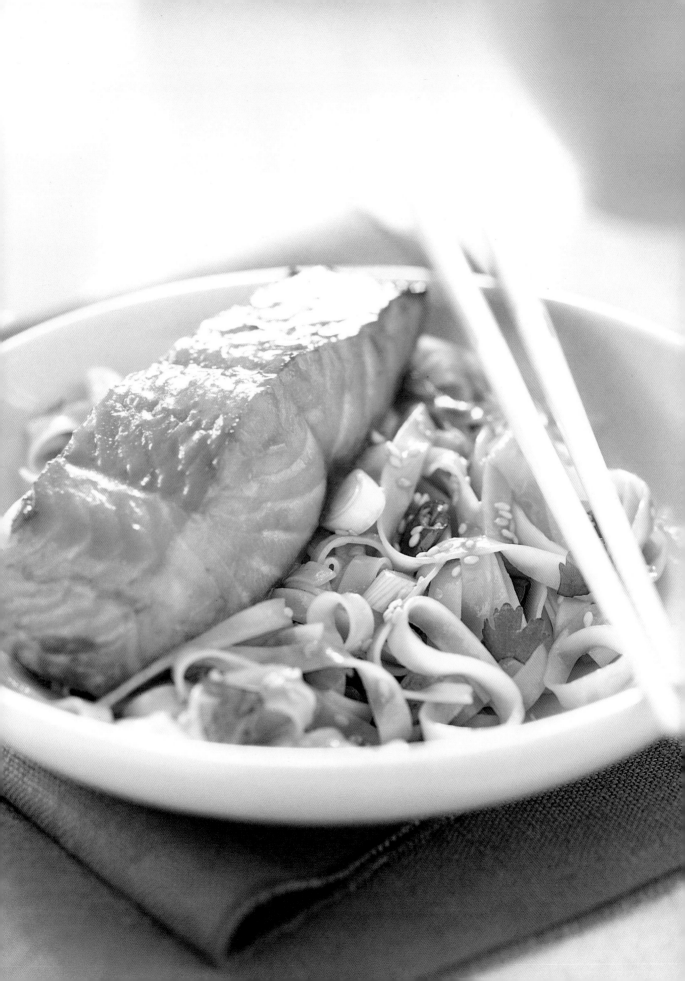

thai beef and noodle salad

250 g (8 oz) piece lean sirloin steak

150 g (5 oz) bean sprouts

1 red pepper, cored, deseeded
and finely sliced

½ cucumber, peeled, deseeded
and sliced

60 g (2½ oz) rocket

200 g (7 oz) dried egg noodles, cooked
according to packet instructions

DRESSING

grated rind and juice of 1 lime

1 tablespoon sesame oil

1 tablespoon Thai fish sauce

1 red chilli, deseeded and finely sliced

4 tablespoons chopped coriander
leaves

1 Heat a griddle or frying pan until very hot. Add the steak and fry for 1–2 minutes on each side, depending how you prefer your meat cooked. Remove from the heat and leave to rest for about 5 minutes.

2 Toss the bean sprouts, red pepper, cucumber and rocket with the noodles.

3 Mix together the dressing ingredients, pour over the salad and combine well. Divide between 4 plates.

4 Slice the steak into thin strips and place on top of the individual salads, then serve.

NUTRITIONAL FACTS

GI rating: LOW

- Kcals – 317
- Protein – 18 g
- Carbohydrate – 40 g
- Fat – 10 g

NUTRITIONAL TIP

Lean red meat is low in fat and calories; it is also a good source of iron.

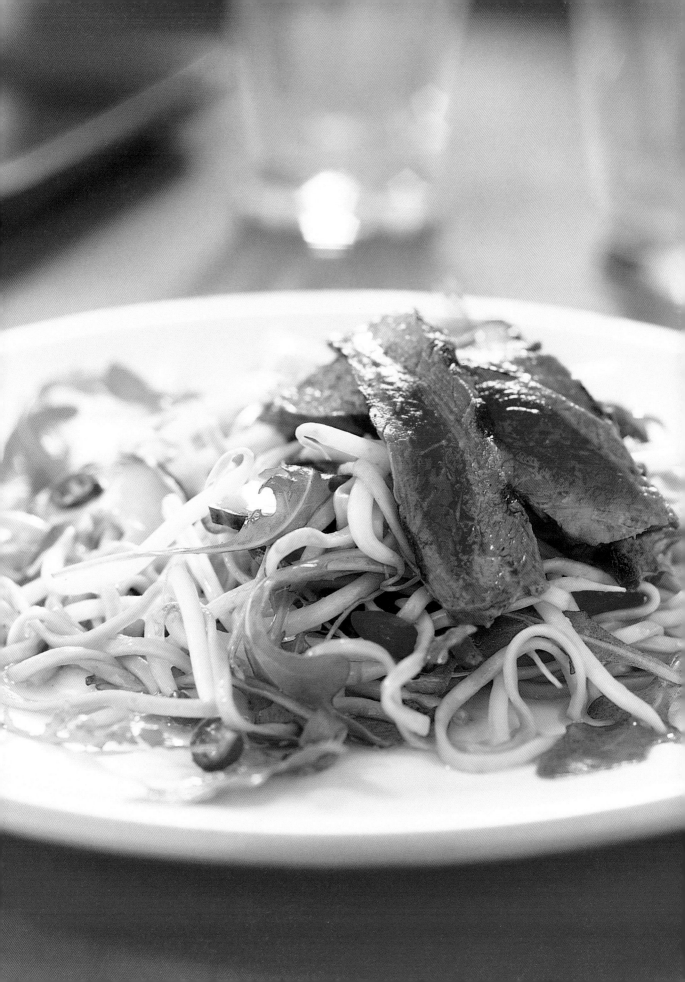

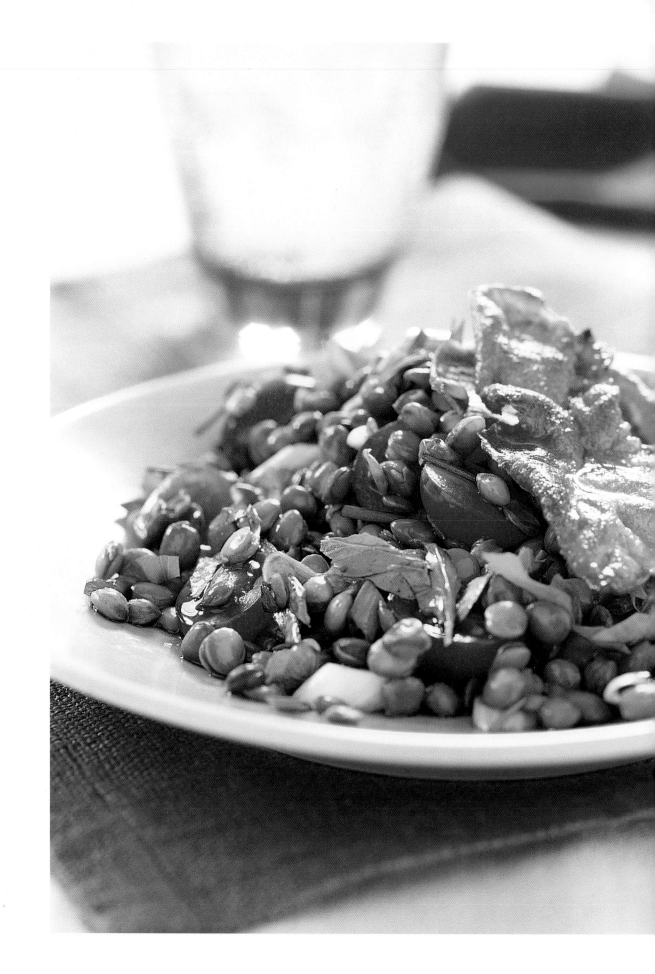

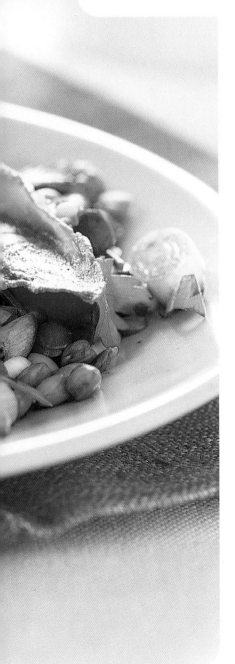

beans, seeds and pulses

3

Peas, beans and lentils all have a low glycaemic index of less than 50. They are high in protein and fibre and low in fat. They are ideal ingredients for vegetarian meals but can be used to lower the glycaemic index of everyone's diet.

Most pulses and beans are available dried or canned. Canned varieties may have a slightly higher glycaemic index, but are ready for use and are therefore much more convenient. Dried beans and pulses need to be soaked and boiled first, so preparation takes longer.

Pulses and beans can be incorporated in recipes in a variety of ways – in salads, casseroles, loaves and rissoles, and in soups. An exotic feast of chickpeas and spices can be as easy to prepare as beans on toast.

chilli bean soup with avocado salsa

1 tablespoon oil

1 large onion, chopped

2 garlic cloves, crushed

2 red chillies, finely chopped

1 teaspoon ground cumin

½ teaspoon ground cinnamon

2 x 400 g (13 oz) cans kidney beans,
   drained and rinsed

400 g (13 oz) can chopped tomatoes

600 ml (1 pint) vegetable stock

tortillas or flatbread, to serve

SALSA

1 small avocado, peeled and
   finely chopped

2 tomatoes, finely chopped

4 tablespoons chopped coriander
   leaves

½ small red onion, finely chopped

salt and pepper

1 Heat the oil in a large saucepan, add the onion, garlic and chillies and fry for 2–3 minutes until the onion begins to soften.

2 Add the spices and continue to fry for a further minute. Add the kidney beans, tomatoes and stock to the pan, bring to the boil, cover and simmer for 15 minutes.

3 Transfer the soup to a food processor or blender and blend until smooth (it may be easier to do this in batches). Return the soup to the pan and heat through.

4 Meanwhile, mix together all the ingredients for the salsa.

5 Serve the soup topped with a spoonful of salsa, with tortillas or flatbread.

NUTRITIONAL FACTS

 Suitable for vegetarians

GI rating: LOW

O Kcals – 264

O Protein – 12 g

O Carbohydrate – 36 g

O Fat – 8 g

NUTRITIONAL TIP

Avocados are a source of monounsaturated fatty acids.

chicken liver, black-eyed bean and spinach salad

1 Heat the oil in a pan, add the onion and garlic and fry for 2 minutes.

2 Add the chicken livers and fry for 3–4 minutes until just cooked through.

3 Stir in the balsamic vinegar, tomatoes and beans and heat through for a further 2 minutes. Toss through the spinach and serve with crusty bread.

1 tablespoon olive oil

1 onion, sliced

1 garlic clove, crushed

250 g (8 oz) chicken livers, halved

2 tablespoons balsamic vinegar

3 tomatoes, chopped

400 g (13 oz) can black-eyed beans,
   drained and rinsed

225 g (7½ oz) baby leaf spinach

crusty bread, to serve

NUTRITIONAL FACTS

GI rating: LOW

- Kcals – 181
- Protein – 18 g
- Carbohydrate – 17 g
- Fat – 5 g

NUTRITIONAL TIP

Spinach is an excellent source of iron and used as a salad ingredient it provides maximum nutritional value.

herby bean cakes

1 Place the beans in a food processor or blender and blend until almost smooth. Add half of the egg and blend again.

2 Stir in the spring onions, herbs and Stilton. Season to taste with salt and pepper.

3 Shape the mixture into 8 balls, then flatten them slightly with the palm of your hand. Coat the patties in flour, then dip them into the remaining egg, then in the breadcrumbs, to coat them. Place on a lightly oiled baking sheet and drizzle with the oil.

4 Cook in a preheated oven at 200°C (400°F), Gas Mark 6 for 10–15 minutes until golden and piping hot. Garnish with a parsley sprig and serve with a tomato and cucumber salad.

2 x 400 g (13 oz) cans cannellini beans, drained and rinsed
2 eggs, beaten
1 bunch of spring onions, finely chopped
4 tablespoons chopped herbs (such as sage, parsley or thyme)
50 g (2 oz) Stilton cheese, crumbled
4 tablespoons plain flour
50 g (2 oz) fine white breadcrumbs
2 tablespoons oil
salt and pepper
parsley sprig, to garnish
tomato and cucumber salad, to serve

NUTRITIONAL FACTS

 Suitable for vegetarians

GI rating: LOW

○ Kcals – 352
○ Protein – 19 g
○ Carbohydrate – 45 g
○ Fat – 11 g

NUTRITIONAL TIP

Fresh parsley is a good source of vitamin C and iron.

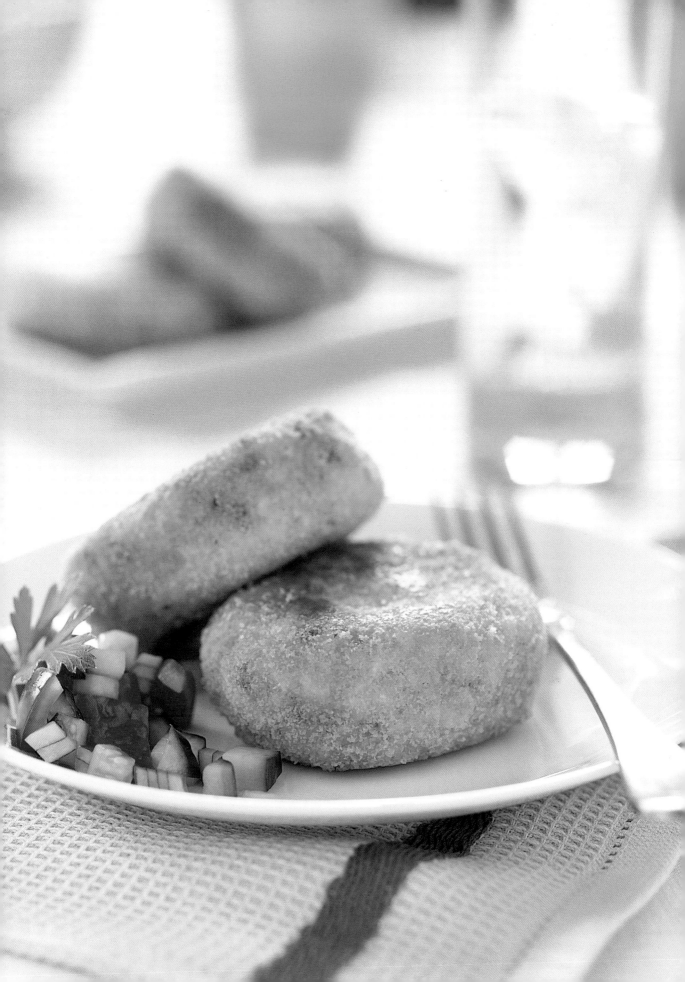

mixed
bean pâté

1 Place all the ingredients in a food processor or blender and blend until almost smooth, but still retaining a little texture.

2 Season to taste with salt and pepper and serve with plenty of crusty bread and a crisp green salad.

2 x 400 g (13 oz) cans mixed beans,
    drained and rinsed
4 tablespoons light crème fraîche
2 tablespoons chopped mixed herbs
    (such as coriander and parsley)
1 tablespoon olive oil
2 tablespoons creamed horseradish
salt and pepper

TO SERVE
crusty bread
green salad

NUTRITIONAL FACTS

(V) Suitable for vegetarians
    GI rating: LOW

- Kcals – 196
- Protein – 11 g
- Carbohydrate – 31 g
- Fat – 10 g

NUTRITIONAL TIP
This quick pâté is a low-fat vegetarian alternative to high fat meat pâtés.

sausage and bean casserole

1 tablespoon oil

1 onion, chopped

1 garlic clove, crushed

1 red pepper, cored, deseeded
    and chopped

4 lean pork sausages, quartered

2 x 400 g (13 oz) cans mixed beans,
    drained and rinsed

400 g (13 oz) can chopped tomatoes

150 ml (¼ pint) vegetable stock

2 tablespoons tomato purée

2 tablespoons chopped parsley

salt and pepper

1 Heat the oil in a saucepan, add the onion, garlic and pepper and fry for 2–3 minutes until beginning to soften.

2 Add the sausages and continue to cook for 5 minutes until browned all over.

3 Lightly crush half of the beans with the back of a fork and add to the pan with the remaining beans, tomatoes, vegetable stock and tomato purée. Season to taste with salt and pepper. Bring to the boil and simmer for 10 minutes. Take off the heat, stir in the parsley and serve.

NUTRITIONAL FACTS

GI rating: LOW

- Kcals – 342
- Protein – 20 g
- Carbohydrate – 38 g
- Fat – 13 g

NUTRITIONAL TIP

Add a carbohydrate such as mashed potato to make this a complete meal.

pan-fried lamb with spiced flageolet beans

½ teaspoon ground cumin

½ teaspoon ground coriander

pinch of chilli powder

1 tablespoon oil

4 lean lamb steaks

1 onion, sliced

1 garlic clove, crushed

4 tablespoons lemon juice

400 g (13 oz) can flageolet beans, drained
   and rinsed

1 tablespoon chopped mint

2 tablespoons light crème fraîche

salad leaves or fresh vegetables,
   to serve

1 Mix together the cumin, coriander, chilli and half the oil in a non-metallic bowl. Add the lamb, coat it in the spices and set aside for 10 minutes.

2 Heat the remaining oil in a nonstick pan, add the onion and garlic and fry for 3–4 minutes until softened.

3 Add the lamb and the marinade and fry for 2–3 minutes on each side, or until cooked to your liking.

4 Add the lemon juice, flageolet beans, mint and crème fraîche and simmer for 1 minute until warmed through. Serve with salad leaves or fresh vegetables.

NUTRITIONAL FACTS

GI rating: LOW

- Kcals – 261
- Protein – 26 g
- Carbohydrate – 16 g
- Fat – 12 g

NUTRITIONAL TIP

Serve this dish with an additional carbohydrate such as rice, potato or pasta.

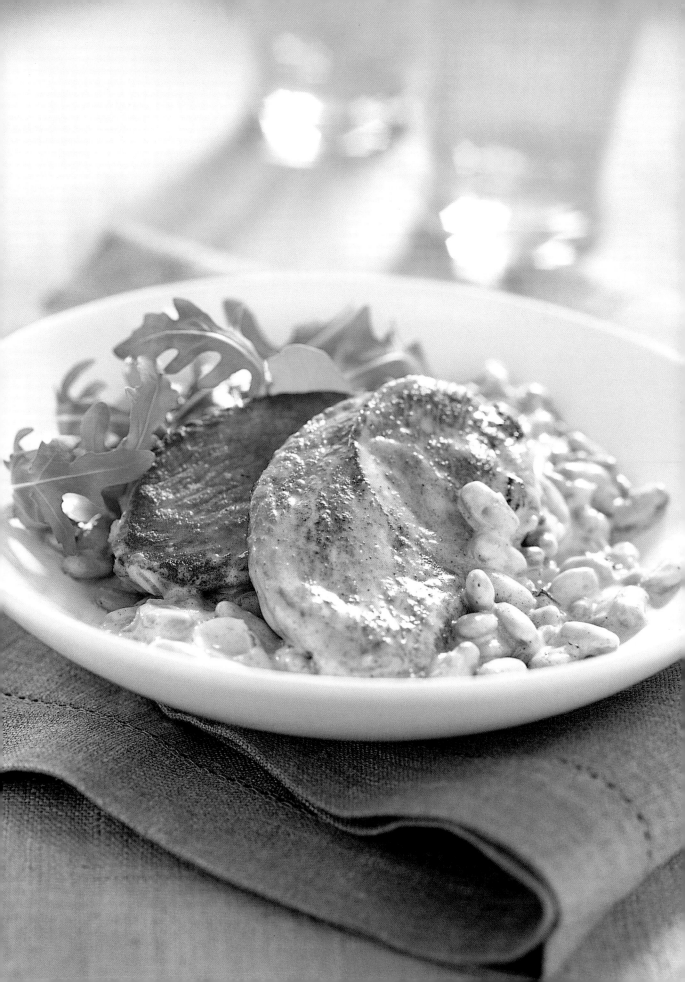

haricot bean and tuna salad

2 x 400 g (13 oz) cans haricot beans,
   drained and rinsed
2 x 200 g (7 oz) cans tuna in water,
   drained
grated rind and juice of 1 lemon
1 tablespoon Dijon mustard
1 teaspoon clear honey
2 tablespoons olive oil
2 tablespoons chopped parsley
salt and pepper

TO SERVE
1 bunch of watercress
crusty bread

1 Tip the beans and tuna into a bowl.

2 In another bowl, mix together the lemon rind and juice, mustard, honey, oil and parsley and season to taste with salt and pepper. Pour the dressing over the beans and tuna, stir well and set aside for 10 minutes to allow the flavours to develop.

3 Serve the salad on a bed of watercress with chunks of crusty bread.

NUTRITIONAL FACTS

GI rating: LOW

- Kcals – 279
- Protein – 32 g
- Carbohydrate – 23 g
- Fat – 6 g

NUTRITIONAL TIP

Canned tuna is available packed in water, brine or oil – choose water to limit your salt and fat intake.

baked trout with butter bean mash

4 trout, about 200 g (7 oz) each

1 lemon, cut into wedges

4 parsley sprigs

1 onion, sliced

salt and pepper

BUTTER BEAN MASH

2 x 400 g (13 oz) cans butter beans,
    drained and rinsed

1 bay leaf

2 garlic cloves

300 ml (½ pint) vegetable stock

2 tablespoons light crème fraîche

1 tablespoon horseradish sauce

1 Cut 4 pieces of kitchen foil big enough to wrap around the fish. Place a trout in the centre of each piece of foil with a couple of lemon wedges, a sprig of parsley and some onion. Season with salt and pepper, then wrap to enclose the fish completely.

2 Bake in a preheated oven at 200°C (400°F), Gas Mark 6 for 15–20 minutes, or until cooked through.

3 Meanwhile, place the butter beans, bay leaf, garlic and vegetable stock in a pan and simmer for 10 minutes. Drain the beans and remove the bay leaf.

4 Mash the bean mixture, crème fraîche and horseradish until smooth. Season to taste with salt and pepper. Remove the fish from the parcels and serve with the mash.

NUTRITIONAL FACTS

GI rating: LOW

- Kcals – 379
- Protein – 48 g
- Carbohydrate – 22 g
- Fat – 12 g

NUTRITIONAL TIP

For extra carbohydrate serve with bread or potatoes.

herby lentil salad with parma ham crisps

1 Heat the oil in a nonstick saucepan, add the garlic and spring onions and fry for 2 minutes.

2 Stir in the lentils, vinegar, herbs and tomatoes and set aside.

3 Heat a frying pan until hot, add the Parma ham and cook for 1–2 minutes, until crisp. Arrange the lentil salad on a large serving dish, place the ham on top and serve.

2 tablespoons olive oil

1 garlic clove, crushed

4 spring onions, sliced

2 x 400 g (13 oz) cans green lentils, drained and rinsed

2 tablespoons balsamic vinegar

3 tablespoons chopped herbs (such as parsley, oregano or basil)

125 g (4 oz) cherry tomatoes, halved

85 g (3¼ oz) sliced Parma ham

NUTRITIONAL FACTS

GI rating: LOW

- Kcals – 262
- Protein – 19 g
- Carbohydrate – 26 g
- Fat – 9 g

NUTRITIONAL TIP

Lentils are a good source of protein and iron, as well as containing isoflavones which may relieve menopausal symptoms.

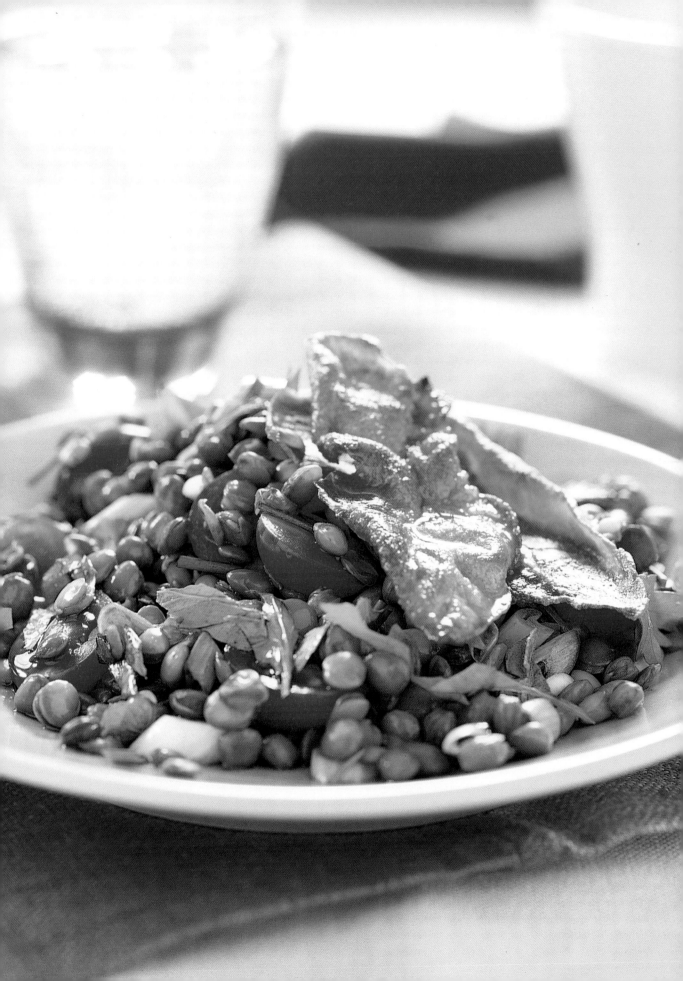

channa chat (mixed bean salad)

1 Mix together all the ingredients in a bowl. Garnish with a sprinkling of garam masala and serve with plain yogurt, if liked.

400 g (13 oz) can chickpeas, drained
   and rinsed

400 g (13 oz) cooked new potatoes,
   quartered

400 g (13 oz) can black-eyed beans,
   drained and rinsed

3 tablespoons sweetcorn kernels,
   defrosted if frozen

1/4 teaspoon salt

1/4 teaspoon chilli powder, or to taste

1/2 green chilli, deseeded and chopped

1/4 teaspoon chat masala

1 tablespoon lemon juice

1 small onion, finely chopped

1 tomato, finely chopped

1/2 teaspoon garam masala, to garnish

plain yogurt, to serve (optional)

NUTRITIONAL FACTS

 Suitable for vegetarians

GI rating: LOW

- Kcals – 270
- Protein – 14 g
- Carbohydrate – 48 g
- Fat – 3 g

NUTRITIONAL TIP

Chickpeas are high energy pulses; they are also rich in carbohydrate and protein and low in fat.

spiced chickpeas in pittas

1 tablespoon oil

2 onions, sliced

2 garlic cloves, crushed

2 tablespoons medium curry paste

6 tomatoes, chopped

2 x 400 g (13 oz) cans chickpeas, drained
   and rinsed

200 g (7 oz) frozen peas, defrosted

2 tablespoons chopped coriander
   leaves

4 pitta breads

4 tablespoons Greek yogurt

1 Heat the oil in a nonstick saucepan. Add the onion and garlic and fry for 4–5 minutes, until softened.

2 Stir in the curry paste and continue to fry for 1 minute. Add the tomatoes and chickpeas and simmer for 10 minutes.

3 Add the peas and coriander and simmer for a further minute.

4 Warm the pittas under a hot grill and serve stuffed with the chickpea mixture and the yogurt.

NUTRITIONAL FACTS

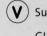 Suitable for vegetarians

GI rating: LOW

- Kcals – 524
- Protein – 24 g
- Carbohydrate – 79 g
- Fat – 15 g

NUTRITIONAL TIP

Tomatoes are very good for you, they are rich in lycopene, which is a potent antioxidant thought to help protect against some forms of cancer.

mini
falafel salad

1 Place two-thirds of the chickpeas in a food processor or blender with the ground coriander, cumin and garlic and blend until almost smooth. Stir in the coriander leaves and the egg yolk.

2 Form the mixture into 16 small balls and brush with the oil. Place under a preheated hot grill and grill for 3–4 minutes until golden.

3 Divide the lettuce, cucumber, the remaining chickpeas and the falafel between 4 plates.

4 Mix together the dressing ingredients. Serve the falafel salad with the dressing and the pitta breads.

2 x 400 g (13 oz) cans chickpeas, drained
    and rinsed
2 teaspoons ground coriander
2 teaspoons ground cumin
2 garlic cloves, crushed
2 tablespoons chopped coriander
    leaves
1 egg yolk, beaten
2 tablespoons oil
toasted mini pitta breads, to serve

SALAD

3 Little Gem lettuces, torn into
    bite-sized pieces
½ cucumber, sliced

DRESSING

300 g (10 oz) plain yogurt
3 tablespoons chopped mint
3 tablespoons chopped parsley
salt and pepper

NUTRITIONAL FACTS

(V) Suitable for vegetarians

GI rating: LOW

O Kcals – 285

O Protein – 15 g

O Carbohydrate – 31 g

O Fat – 11 g

NUTRITIONAL TIP

Falafel are generally fried in oil; these mini falafel are lower in fat as they are brushed with oil and baked. Serve with the yogurt dressing, which is low in fat, high in protein and rich in vitamins.

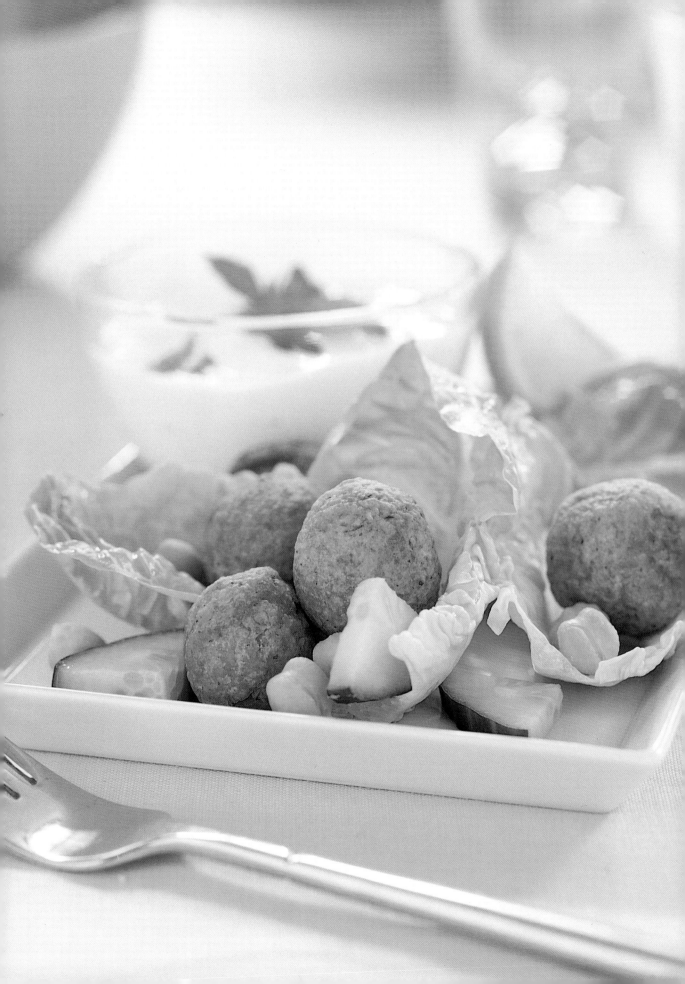

moroccan tomato and chickpea salad

1 Simply mix together all the ingredients in a large non-metallic bowl, set aside for 10 minutes to allow the flavours to infuse, then serve.

1 red onion, finely sliced

2 x 400 g (13 oz) cans chickpeas, drained and rinsed

4 tomatoes, chopped

4 tablespoons lemon juice

1 tablespoon olive oil

handful of herbs (such as mint and parsley), chopped

pinch of paprika

pinch of ground cumin

salt and pepper

NUTRITIONAL FACTS

 Suitable for vegetarians

GI rating: LOW

- Kcals – 200
- Protein – 12 g
- Carbohydrate – 30 g
- Fat – 5 g

NUTRITIONAL TIP

Red onions are a good source of flavonols which act as antioxidants.

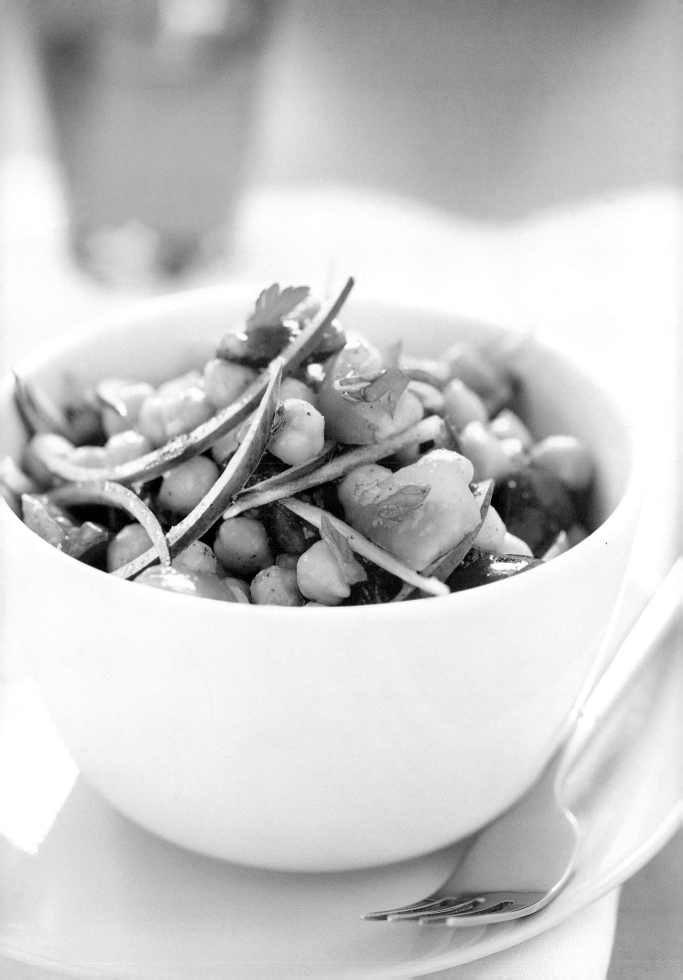

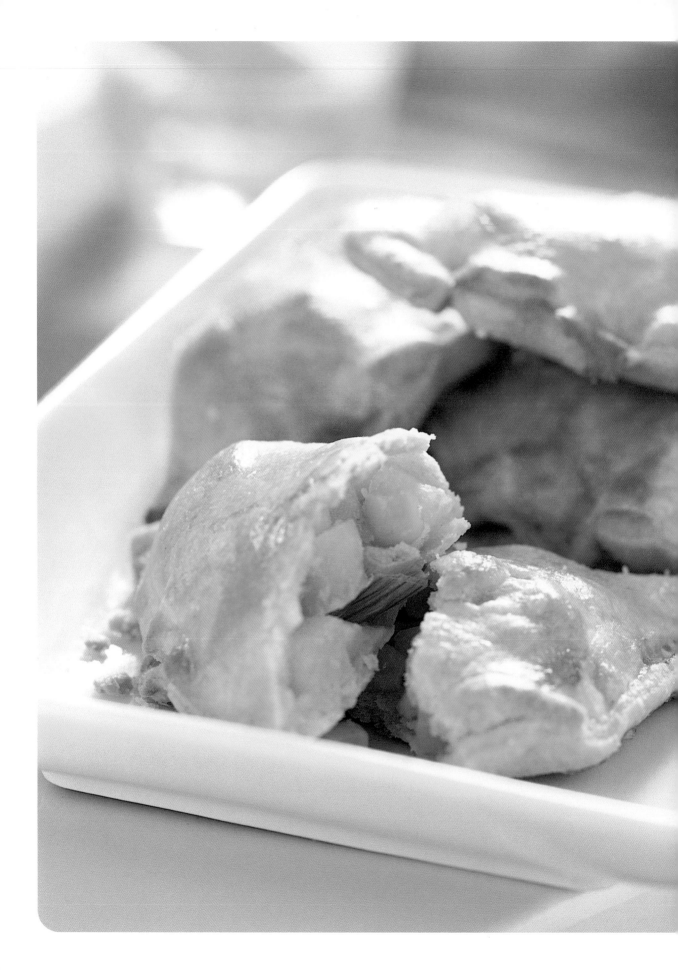

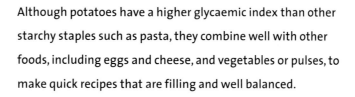

eat more potatoes

4

Although potatoes have a higher glycaemic index than other starchy staples such as pasta, they combine well with other foods, including eggs and cheese, and vegetables or pulses, to make quick recipes that are filling and well balanced.

New potatoes tend to have a lower glycaemic index than old potatoes, and cold potatoes tend to have a lower glycaemic index than those served hot. Mashed potatoes combine well with foods which have a lower glycaemic index, such as beans, peas and pulses.

As an alternative, try sweet potatoes in recipes – they are higher in fibre, have a lower glycaemic index than normal potatoes, and make a pleasant change.

all-day breakfast

4 lean back bacon rashers, halved
    lengthways
4 good-quality sausages, halved
    lengthways
400 g (13 oz) new potatoes, cooked
    and halved
16 mushrooms, sliced
4 tomatoes, halved
4 eggs
pepper
crusty wholegrain bread, to serve

1 Heat a large nonstick frying pan and add the bacon and sausages. Fry for 2–3 minutes.

2 Add the potatoes and continue to fry for 3–4 minutes until beginning to brown. Add the mushrooms and tomatoes and continue to fry for 1–2 minutes. Drain off any excess fat and spread out all the ingredients in the pan.

3 Crack the eggs into the pan and allow to run across the base of the pan. (If your pan is not big enough, then you could cook this in two batches.)

4 Cook for a further minute or until the eggs are done to your liking. Season to taste with pepper and serve with chunks of crusty wholegrain bread.

NUTRITIONAL FACTS

GI rating: LOW–MEDIUM

- Kcals – 326
- Protein – 20 g
- Carbohydrate – 21 g
- Fat – 15 g

NUTRITIONAL TIP

Avoid adding any oil to the pan to minimize the amount of fat in this recipe.

leek and potato soup

1 tablespoon olive oil

1 onion, chopped

500 g (1 lb) leeks, finely sliced

500 g (1 lb) potatoes, chopped

1 litre (1¾ pints) vegetable stock

2 tablespoons light crème fraîche

¼ teaspoon grated nutmeg

salt and pepper

1 Heat the oil in a saucepan, add the onion and fry for 2–3 minutes. Add the leeks and potatoes and cook for 5 minutes.

2 Add the stock, bring to the boil and simmer for 15 minutes, until the potatoes are tender.

3 Transfer to a food processor or blender and blend until smooth. Stir in the crème fraîche and nutmeg and season to taste with salt and plenty of black pepper.

NUTRITIONAL FACTS

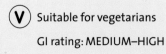 Suitable for vegetarians

GI rating: MEDIUM–HIGH

- Kcals – 159
- Protein – 5 g
- Carbohydrate – 28 g
- Fat – 5 g

NUTRITIONAL TIP

Leeks and other members of the onion family are a good source of sulphur-containing phytochemicals, which help to protect against heart disease.

spring onion and potato pasties

375 g (12 oz) ready-made shortcrust pastry

plain flour, for dusting

a little milk, for brushing

FILLING

1 medium potato, cut into small cubes

4 spring onions, sliced

45 g (1¾ oz) sweetcorn kernels, defrosted if frozen

2 tablespoons light crème fraîche

salt and pepper

1 Roll out the pastry on a lightly floured work surface to a thickness of 3 mm (⅛ inch). Using a saucer, cut out 12 rounds of pastry, 12 cm (5 inches) in diameter.

2 Cook the potatoes for 5 minutes in boiling water, then drain. Mix with the spring onions, sweetcorn and crème fraîche and season to taste with salt and pepper then place a little of the mixture in the centre of each piece of pastry.

3 Dampen the edges of the pastry with a little water and fold in half to cover the filling.

4 Press down the edges with a fork, then place on a greased baking sheet. Brush with a little milk, then cook in a preheated oven at 200°C (400°F), Gas Mark 6 for 15–20 minutes until golden brown.

NUTRITIONAL FACTS

 Suitable for vegetarians

GI rating: MEDIUM

- Kcals – 216
- Protein – 3 g
- Carbohydrate – 25 g
- Fat – 13 g

NUTRITIONAL TIP

Pastry is high in fat, so roll it out thinly and use a single crust where possible.

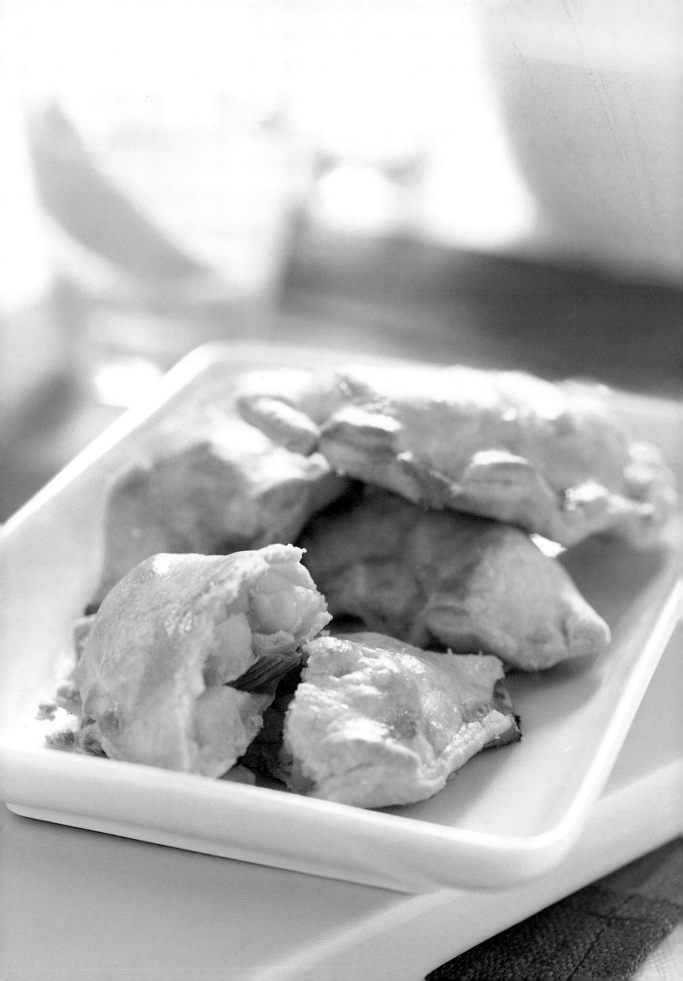

potatoes with garlic and pancetta

125 g (4 oz) cubed pancetta

1 onion, chopped

625 g (1¼ lb) potatoes, cooked
  and cubed

2 garlic cloves, crushed

1 tablespoon chopped parsley

2 tablespoons grated Parmesan cheese

1 Cook the pancetta in a nonstick frying pan for 3–4 minutes until beginning to brown.

2 Add the onion, potatoes and garlic and continue to fry for 8–10 minutes until the potatoes are browned, then stir in the parsley.

3 Place the mixture in a flameproof dish and sprinkle over the Parmesan. Cook under a preheated hot grill for 1–2 minutes, until the Parmesan is melted and golden.

NUTRITIONAL FACTS

GI rating: MEDIUM–HIGH

- Kcals – 246
- Protein – 13 g
- Carbohydrate – 28 g
- Fat – 8 g

NUTRITIONAL TIP

Eating a garlic clove a day is thought to be beneficial in promoting a healthy heart and lowering cholesterol.

smoked mackerel and potato salad

1 kg (2 lb) baby new potatoes, halved

4 tablespoons fat-free French dressing

1 punnet mustard and cress, chopped

1 avocado, stoned and chopped

3 spring onions, sliced

2 peppered smoked mackerel
   fillets, flaked

1 Cook the potatoes until tender. Drain, then toss them in the dressing and leave to cool for 10 minutes.

2 When the potatoes are cool, gently stir in the mustard and cress, avocado, spring onions and smoked mackerel and serve.

NUTRITIONAL FACTS

GI rating: MEDIUM

- Kcals – 289
- Protein – 9 g
- Carbohydrate – 20 g
- Fat – 18 g

NUTRITIONAL TIP

Avocados are high in monounsaturated fats, which are thought to lower blood cholesterol levels.

crushed new potatoes with herby salmon

750 g (1½ lb) new potatoes

knob of butter

grated rind and juice of 2 limes

1 bunch of spring onions, sliced

4 pieces boneless, skinless salmon
   fillet, about 125 g (4 oz) each

4 tablespoons light crème fraîche

3 tablespoons chopped mixed herbs
   (such as parsley and dill)

salt and pepper

lime wedges, to garnish

1 Cook the potatoes in a pan of lightly salted boiling water until tender. Drain and lightly crush with a fork.

2 Stir in the butter, half of the lime rind and juice, and half of the spring onions and season with plenty of black pepper.

3 Place the salmon pieces on a foil-lined grill pan and cook under a preheated moderate grill for 6–7 minutes, turning halfway through cooking, or until the salmon is just cooked.

4 Mix together the remaining lime rind and juice, spring onions, crème fraîche and herbs. Serve the salmon with the potatoes and the herby sauce, garnished with lime wedges.

NUTRITIONAL FACTS

GI rating: MEDIUM

- Kcals – 350
- Protein – 45 g
- Carbohydrate – 31 g
- Fat – 8 g

NUTRITIONAL TIP

Potatoes are high in carbohydrates, protein and fibre and are therefore very good for you. It is a myth that they are fattening; it is only when they are cooked in oil or have cream and butter added that they become so.

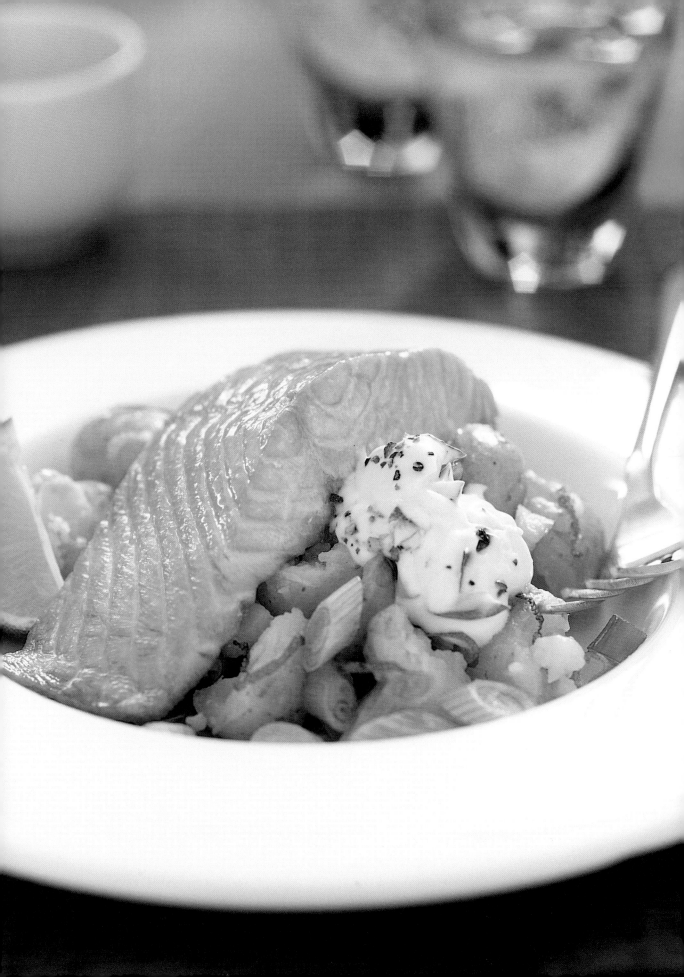

salmon fishcakes with tomato and pepper salsa

500 g (1 lb) potatoes, chopped

grated rind and juice of 1 lemon

4 tablespoons milk

1 bunch of spring onions, sliced

½ teaspoon cayenne pepper

2 x 200 g (7 oz) cans salmon in water or
  brine, drained and flaked

2 tablespoons plain flour

1 egg, beaten

100 g (3½ oz) fresh white breadcrumbs

1 tablespoon olive oil

salt and pepper

SALSA

4 tomatoes, finely chopped

1 green chilli, finely chopped

1 red pepper, cored, deseeded and
  finely chopped

grated rind and juice of 1 lime

2 tablespoons chopped parsley

1 Cook the potatoes in a pan of lightly salted boiling water until tender. Drain and mash.

2 Stir in the lemon rind and juice, milk, spring onions, cayenne pepper and the salmon. Season to taste with salt and pepper.

3 Form the mixture into 8 patties. Dip them in flour, then the egg and then the breadcrumbs.

4 Place on a lightly oiled baking sheet, and drizzle over the remaining oil. Cook in a preheated oven at 200°C (400°F), Gas Mark 6, for 12–15 minutes until golden and piping hot.

5 Meanwhile, mix together all the salsa ingredients. Serve the salsa with the fishcakes.

NUTRITIONAL FACTS

GI rating: MEDIUM

- Kcals – 385
- Protein – 25 g
- Carbohydrate – 46 g
- Fat – 12 g

NUTRITIONAL TIP

Red and orange fruit and vegetables are a good source of beta-carotene. This is an antioxidant that can protect against heart disease.

hearty
seafood soup

1 Melt the butter in a large saucepan, add the onion, bay leaf, celery and potatoes and fry for 3–4 minutes.

2 Add the milk and fish stock, bring to the boil, cover and simmer for 15–20 minutes, until the potatoes are cooked.

3 Add the fish, prawns, peas and sweetcorn to the pan and continue to simmer for a further 5 minutes or until the fish is cooked through.

4 Season with salt and pepper, turn into a warmed tureen and top with the parsley and the chopped tomato. Serve with bread.

15 g (½ oz) butter

1 onion, chopped

1 bay leaf

2 celery sticks, finely sliced

300 g (10 oz) floury potatoes, cubed

450 ml (¾ pint) skimmed milk

450 ml (¾ pint) fish stock

375 g (12 oz) mixed boneless, skinless
    fish fillets (such as smoked haddock,
    cod and salmon), cubed

100 g (3½ oz) cooked peeled prawns

100 g (3½ oz) frozen peas

100 g (3½ oz) frozen sweetcorn kernels

3 tablespoons chopped parsley

2 tomatoes, finely chopped

bread, to serve

NUTRITIONAL FACTS

GI rating: MEDIUM

- Kcals – 301
- Protein – 30 g
- Carbohydrate – 30 g
- Fat – 7 g

NUTRITIONAL TIP

Try to use unsaturated fat for cooking. Butter may be used in small amounts where flavour is important.

lemon chicken with potato wedges and garlic

1 Cut 3 slits in each chicken breast, then place them in an ovenproof dish with the potatoes and garlic.

2 Mix together the lemon rind and juice, olive oil and stock. Season with salt and pepper and pour over the chicken and potatoes.

3 Cover the dish with foil and bake in a preheated oven at 200°C (400°F), Gas Mark 6, for 25 minutes. Remove the foil and continue to cook for 5 minutes more.

4 When the chicken and potatoes are cooked through, sprinkle with the oregano and serve.

4 boneless, skinless chicken breasts

500 g (1 lb) potatoes, cut into wedges
    and parboiled

4 garlic cloves

grated rind and juice of 1 lemon

1 tablespoon olive oil

150 ml (¼ pint) chicken stock

2 tablespoons chopped oregano

salt and pepper

NUTRITIONAL FACTS

GI rating: MEDIUM–HIGH

- Kcals – 304
- Protein – 43 g
- Carbohydrate – 20 g
- Fat – 5 g

NUTRITIONAL TIP

Use reduced-salt stock cubes or make your own stock to cut down on the amount of salt in your diet.

mediterranean potato salad

1 Cook the potatoes in a saucepan of lightly salted boiling water until tender. Drain, then stir in the dressing and add the sun-dried tomatoes.

2 Leave the potatoes to cool for 10 minutes. Stir in the olives, red onion, feta and herbs and toss well. Serve warm.

1 kg (2 lb) small new potatoes

4 tablespoons fat-free French dressing

4 sun-dried tomatoes in oil, sliced

50 g (2 oz) black olives, pitted

1 red onion, finely sliced

50 g (2 oz) feta cheese, cubed

large bunch of herbs (such as parsley or basil), chopped

NUTRITIONAL FACTS

 Suitable for vegetarians

GI rating: MEDIUM

○ Kcals – 266

○ Protein – 7 g

○ Carbohydrate – 44 g

○ Fat – 8 g

NUTRITIONAL TIP

Olives and sun-dried tomatoes contain oil and salt, but you only need to use a small amount for a rich flavour.

pan-fried calves liver with mustard and sage mash

750 g (1½ lb) potatoes, cubed

2 garlic cloves

6 tablespoons light crème fraîche

1 tablespoon chopped sage

4 slices of calves liver, about 150 g
  (5 oz) each

2 tablespoons seasoned flour

1 tablespoon olive oil

salt and pepper

gravy, to serve

1 Cook the potatoes and garlic in a saucepan of lightly salted boiling water for 10–12 minutes until tender, then drain.

2 Mash the potatoes and garlic with the crème fraîche and sage and season to taste with plenty of freshly ground black pepper.

3 Meanwhile, press the pieces of liver into the seasoned flour to coat them all over. Heat the oil in a nonstick frying pan, add the liver and fry for 1–2 minutes each side or until cooked to your liking. Serve with the mash and gravy.

NUTRITIONAL FACTS

GI rating: HIGH

- Kcals – 307
- Protein – 31 g
- Carbohydrate – 30 g
- Fat – 12 g

NUTRITIONAL TIP

Liver is a good source of fat-soluble vitamin A, however you should avoid it if you are pregnant as excess vitamin A can be harmful to an unborn baby.

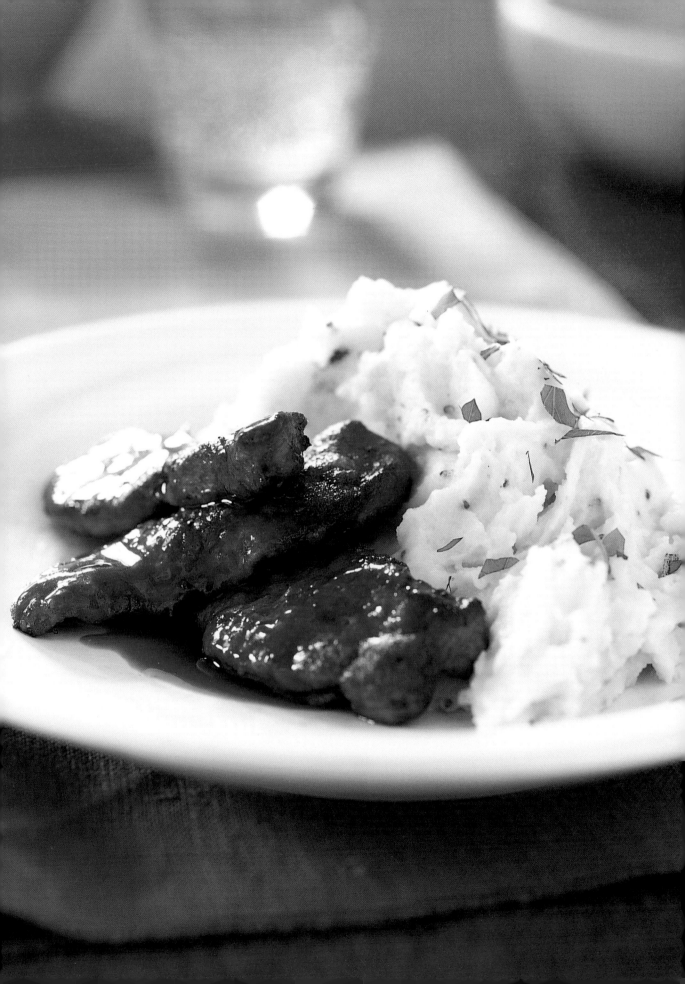

tenderloin of pork with pear and potato

500 g (1 lb) piece pork tenderloin

2 garlic cloves, cut into slivers

1 tablespoon seasoned flour

1 tablespoon oil

150 ml (¼ pint) dry cider

500 g (1 lb) new potatoes, parboiled

2 pears, quartered and cored

2 thyme sprigs

3 tablespoons light crème fraîche

salt and pepper

steamed vegetables or salad, to serve

1 Make a few small cuts in the pork with a sharp knife and push a sliver of garlic into each cut. Rub the pork all over with the seasoned flour.

2 Heat the oil in a frying pan, add the pork and fry for 3–4 minutes over a moderate heat until browned on all sides. Add the cider and simmer until reduced by half.

3 Transfer the pork and juices to a shallow ovenproof dish with the potatoes, pears and thyme.

4 Place in a preheated oven at 200°C (400°F), Gas Mark 6 for 20 minutes or until the pork is cooked through and the potatoes are tender. Stir the crème fraîche through the cooking juices and season to taste with salt and pepper. Serve with steamed vegetables or salad.

NUTRITIONAL FACTS

GI rating: MEDIUM

- Kcals – 430
- Protein – 43 g
- Carbohydrate – 42 g
- Fat – 12 g

NUTRITIONAL TIP

Choose a lean piece of pork which is low in fat and remove any visible fat before cooking.

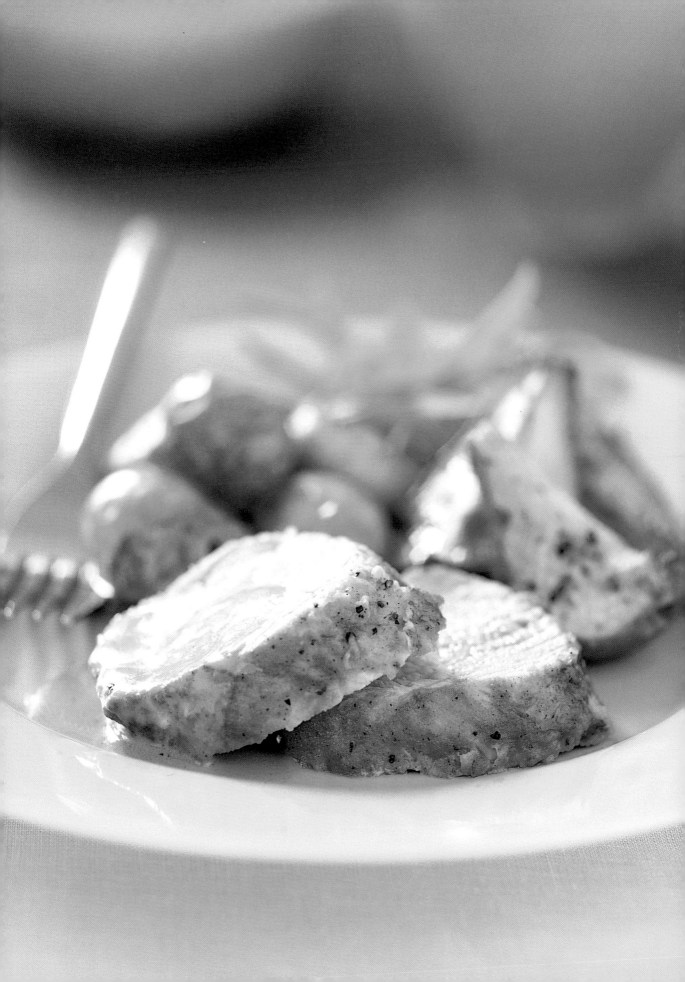

minted lamb with potato rosti

8 lean lamb cutlets

1 garlic clove, crushed

1 teaspoon olive oil

1 tablespoon mint sauce

1 teaspoon clear honey

red cabbage, to serve

chopped mint, to garnish

ROSTI

750 g (1½ lb) potatoes

1 egg, beaten

1 tablespoon plain flour

1 tablespoon oil

1 Place the lamb cutlets, in one layer, in a non-metallic dish. Mix together the garlic, oil, mint sauce and honey and pour over the lamb. Set aside while preparing the rosti.

2 Boil the potatoes in their skins for 10 minutes. Refresh under cold running water. Grate the potatoes, then mix together with the egg and flour. Divide the potato mixture into 8 portions and pat into little flat cakes.

3 Heat the oil in a frying pan, add the rosti cakes and cook for 2–3 minutes on each side, until golden.

4 Meanwhile, remove the lamb from the marinade, place on a baking tray, brush with a little of the marinade and cook under a preheated hot grill for 2–3 minutes on each side, or until done to your liking. Serve the lamb on the rosti cakes with red cabbage, garnish with chopped mint.

NUTRITIONAL FACTS

GI rating: HIGH

- Kcals – 430
- Protein – 33 g
- Carbohydrate – 32 g
- Fat – 17 g

NUTRITIONAL TIP

Red cabbage is rich in vitamin C, folate, beta-carotene and fibre and makes a great accompaniment to any meal.

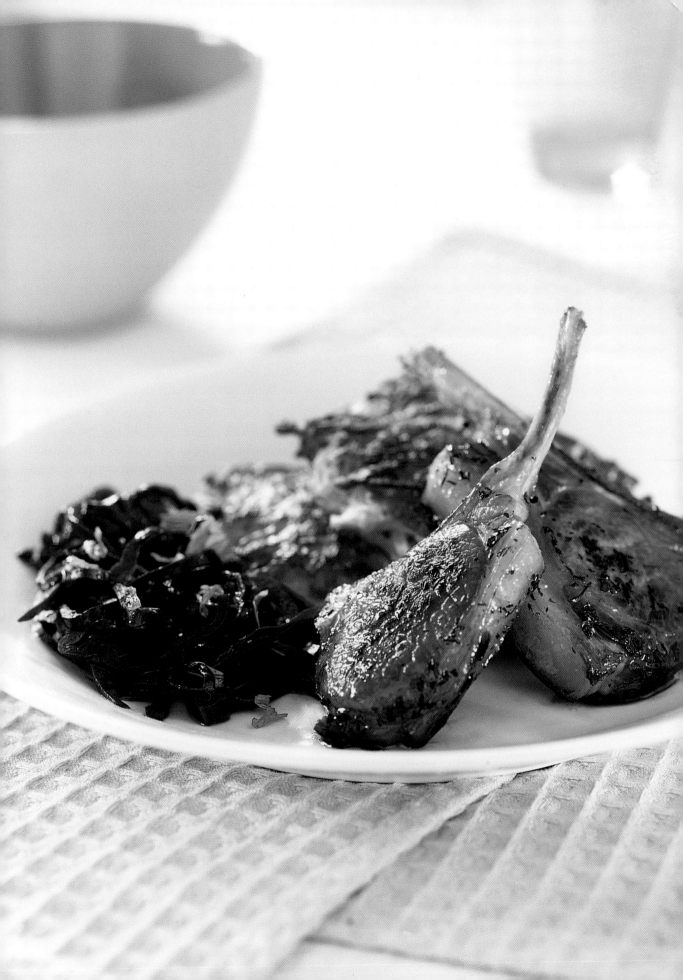

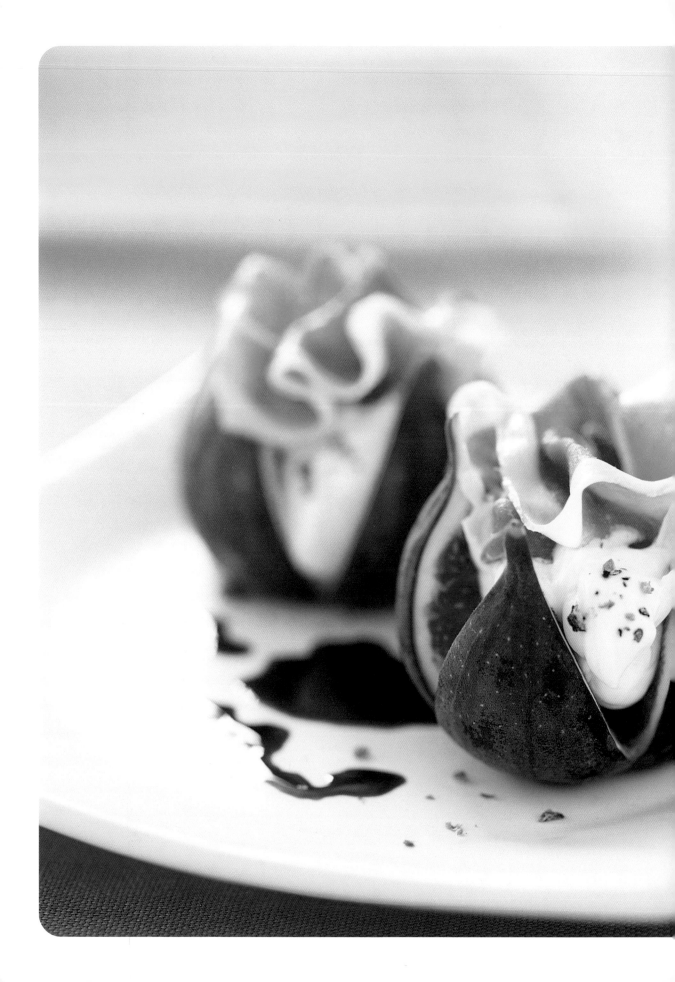

extra fruit and vegetables

5

One simple thing that you can do to improve your diet is to eat more fruit and vegetables. By replacing a proportion of your meal with fruit or vegetables, you can automatically reduce the calories, increase the fibre content and lower the glycaemic index. You also increase your vitamin and mineral intake and reduce your salt intake.

Citrus fruits, such as oranges and grapefruits, have a lower glycaemic index than some tropical fruits, such as pineapple and mango. Canned fruits, such as peaches, can have a lower glycaemic index than their fresh counterparts, so it helps to choose carefully.

Increased acidity is also associated with a lower glycaemic index, as are dried fruits which are high in fibre. The recipes in this section may be used to accompany other dishes, or can be served as vegetarian meals with extra bread, pasta or rice.

Whether you use fresh, frozen, canned or dried fruit and vegetables, aim to include at least five portions every day in your diet.

Preparation time: 10 minutes **Cooking time: 20 minutes**

coconut and butternut squash soup

1 tablespoon olive oil

1 onion, chopped

1 garlic clove, crushed

2 butternut squashes, peeled, deseeded and cubed

2 teaspoons medium curry paste

600 ml (1 pint) vegetable stock

200 ml (7 fl oz) reduced fat coconut milk

2 tablespoons chopped coriander leaves

crusty bread, to serve

1 Heat the oil in a nonstick saucepan. Add the onion and garlic and fry for 4–5 minutes until softened.

2 Add the squash and continue to fry for 1 minute. Stir in the curry paste and fry for a further minute.

3 Pour over the stock, bring to the boil, then cover the pan and simmer for 15 minutes, until the squash is tender.

4 Transfer the soup to a food processor or blender and blend until smooth. Return it to the pan, add the coconut milk and coriander, stir and season to taste with salt and pepper. Heat through, then serve with plenty of crusty bread.

NUTRITIONAL FACTS

 Suitable for vegetarians

GI rating: MEDIUM

- Kcals – 120
- Protein – 2 g
- Carbohydrate – 18 g
- Fat – 4 g

NUTRITIONAL TIP

Butternut squash is a nutritious, starchy root vegetable which can be used as an alternative to potatoes.

bacon, spinach and blue cheese salad

3 smoked back bacon rashers, chopped

25 g (1 oz) pine nuts

225 g (7½ oz) baby spinach leaves

50 g (2 oz) Gorgonzola cheese, cubed

12 cherry tomatoes, halved

crusty bread, to serve

DRESSING

1 teaspoon wholegrain mustard

2 tablespoons balsamic vinegar

1 teaspoon clear honey

1 Fry the bacon in a nonstick frying pan until crisp. Add the pine nuts and continue to cook for 1–2 minutes until the nuts are beginning to brown.

2 Toss together the spinach, Gorgonzola and tomatoes, then stir these into the bacon and pine nuts. Place the salad in a serving bowl.

3 Mix together the dressing ingredients and drizzle over the salad. Serve with crusty bread.

NUTRITIONAL FACTS

GI rating: MEDIUM
- Kcals – 146
- Protein – 8 g
- Carbohydrate – 5 g
- Fat – 16 g

NUTRITIONAL TIP

Although honey is high in sugar it can be used in small amounts in dressings and in cooking to add sweetness and flavour.

warm
aubergine salad

1 Heat the oil in a nonstick frying pan. Add the aubergines and fry for 10 minutes until golden and softened. Add the red onion, capers, tomatoes, parsley and vinegar and stir to combine.

2 Remove the pan from the heat and leave to cool for 10 minutes, then serve with salad leaves and bread.

2 tablespoons olive oil

2 aubergines, cut into small cubes

1 red onion, finely sliced

2 tablespoons capers, roughly chopped

4 tomatoes, chopped

4 tablespoons chopped parsley

1 tablespoon balsamic vinegar

TO SERVE

salad leaves

fresh crusty bread

NUTRITIONAL FACTS

 Suitable for vegetarians

GI rating: LOW

- Kcals – 99
- Protein – 3 g
- Carbohydrate – 9 g
- Fat – 6 g

NUTRITIONAL TIP

The purple colour of aubergine skin is due to a type of anthocyanin, which acts as an antioxidant. The aubergine is also low in calories, however it does soak up oil, so be careful when cooking it.

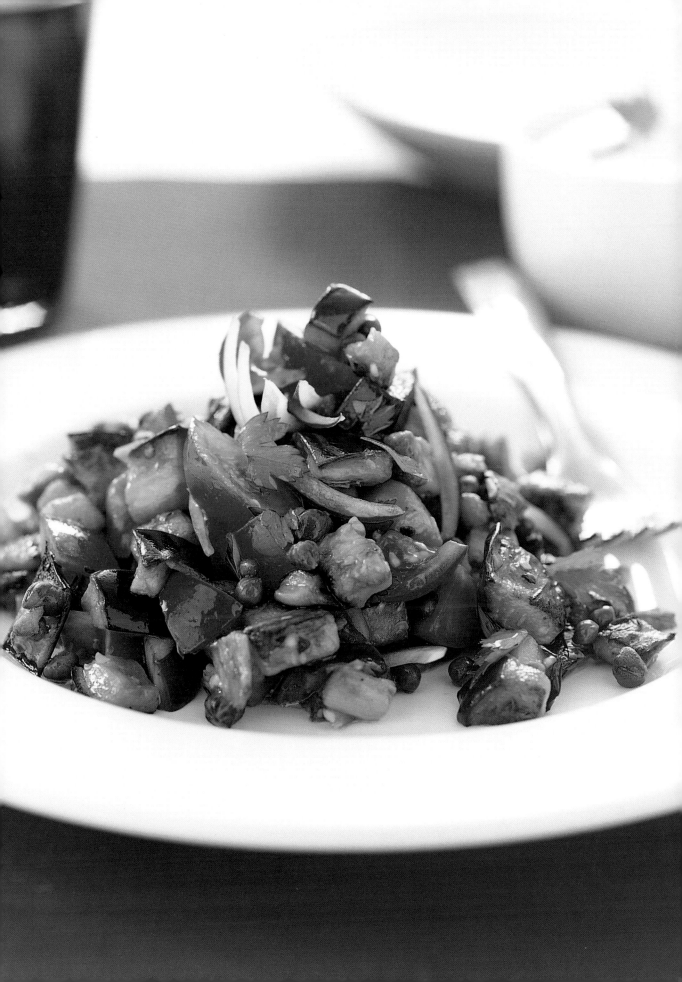

charred asparagus with parmesan

1 Place the asparagus on a baking sheet and drizzle over the oil. Place under a preheated hot grill and cook for 3–4 minutes, turning occasionally, until tender and beginning to char.

2 Serve the asparagus with the Parmesan shavings and plenty of black pepper sprinkled over the top.

250 g (8 oz) asparagus tips

2 teaspoons olive oil

25 g (1 oz) Parmesan cheese shavings

pepper

NUTRITIONAL FACTS

 Suitable for vegetarians

GI rating: LOW–MEDIUM

- Kcals – 93
- Protein – 4 g
- Carbohydrate – 1 g
- Fat – 7 g

NUTRITIONAL TIP

Asparagus is a source of fructo-oligosaccharides (FOS), a type of fibre that promotes the growth of healthy bacteria in the gut.

grilled spiced butternut squash

2 butternut squash, peeled, deseeded
   and cubed
1 tablespoon coriander seeds
1 tablespoon cumin seeds
1 tablespoon paprika
2 tablespoons olive oil
2 tablespoons chopped coriander
   leaves
4 tablespoons Greek yogurt

1 Place the squash in a pan of boiling water and simmer for 5 minutes. Drain and place on a baking sheet.

2 Put the coriander and cumin seeds into a small pan and heat for 1 minute until the spices become fragrant, then crush using a pestle and mortar.

3 Combine the crushed seed mixture, paprika and olive oil. Drizzle over the squash, then place under a preheated hot grill for 8–10 minutes, until tender and beginning to char.

4 Mix together the chopped coriander and yogurt and serve with the spiced squash.

NUTRITIONAL FACTS

 Suitable for vegetarians
GI rating: MEDIUM–HIGH

- Kcals – 155
- Protein – 5 g
- Carbohydrate – 13 g
- Fat – 9 g

NUTRITIONAL TIP
Butternut squash is an excellent source of beta-carotene, which can be converted by the body into vitamin A.

summer vegetable salad

1 Use a vegetable peeler to slice the courgettes and the carrots into fine ribbons. Place them in a pan of boiling water, then immediately drain and refresh under cold running water.

2 Toss the courgette and carrot ribbons with the mangetout, red pepper, bean sprouts, chilli, coriander, sesame seeds, oil and lime rind and juice and set aside for 20 minutes to allow the flavours to infuse. Serve in a large bowl.

2 courgettes

2 carrots

150 g (5 oz) mangetout, halved
   lengthways

1 red pepper, cored, deseeded and sliced

150 g (5 oz) bean sprouts

1 red chilli, finely sliced

4 tablespoons chopped coriander
   leaves

2 tablespoons sesame seeds, toasted

1 tablespoon sesame oil

grated rind and juice of 1 lime

NUTRITIONAL FACTS

 Suitable for vegetarians

GI rating: MEDIUM

- Kcals – 116
- Protein – 5 g
- Carbohydrate – 7 g
- Fat – 7 g

NUTRITIONAL TIP

Chillies owe their heat to the phytochemical capsaicin, which is concentrated in the seeds and can help relieve nasal congestion. They are also rich in vitamin C.

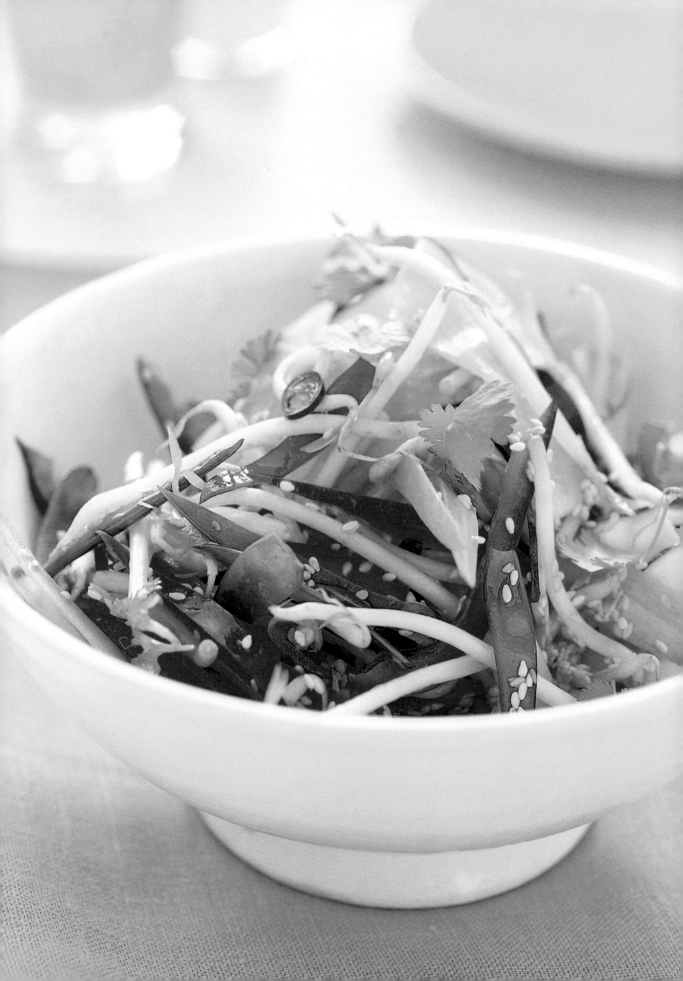

garlic mushrooms with wilted spinach and crispy bacon

1 Place the mushrooms, gill sides up, in a large nonstick frying pan with the water.

2 Mix together the cream cheese and lemon rind, then season to taste with salt and pepper. Divide the mixture between the mushroom caps. Cover and cook over a low heat for 5–6 minutes.

3 Layer the spinach over the mushrooms, cover and continue to cook for 2 minutes, until the spinach has wilted.

4 Divide the mushrooms between warmed serving plates, then top with the bacon and serve.

8 open-cap mushrooms

4 tablespoons water

200 g (7 oz) extra-light garlic and herb
  cream cheese

grated rind of 1 lemon

100 g (3½ oz) baby leaf spinach

4 lean back bacon rashers, grilled until
  crisp, then roughly chopped

NUTRITIONAL FACTS

GI rating: LOW

- Kcals – 93
- Protein – 5 g
- Carbohydrate – 0 g
- Fat – 8 g

NUTRITIONAL TIP

Look out for the different levels of fat in soft cheese – extra-light is low fat and light is medium-fat.

aubergine and mozzarella stacks with pesto dressing

2 aubergines, each sliced into 12 rounds

1 tablespoon olive oil

16 basil leaves

4 tomatoes, each sliced into 4

150 g (5 oz) mozzarella cheese, cut into 8 slices

rocket leaves, to serve

DRESSING

1 tablespoon pesto

1 tablespoon balsamic vinegar

1 Brush the aubergine slices with a little oil. Place them on a grill pan and cook under a preheated hot grill for 2–3 minutes on each side until beginning to brown.

2 Place 8 slices of aubergine on a baking sheet and top each one with a basil leaf, a slice of tomato and a slice of mozzarella. Place another piece of aubergine on top of each stack, then another slice of tomato, a basil leaf and finally another slice of aubergine.

3 Cook in a preheated oven at 200°C (400°F), Gas Mark 6, for 15 minutes, until golden and tender.

4 Mix together the dressing ingredients. Serve the aubergine stacks on a bed of rocket, and drizzle with the dressing.

NUTRITIONAL FACTS

 Suitable for vegetarians

GI rating: MEDIUM

- Kcals – 157
- Protein – 7 g
- Carbohydrate – 9 g
- Fat – 10 g

NUTRITIONAL TIP

As well as being one of the most popular of salad vegetables, tomatoes are a source of vitamins C and E, potassium and beta-carotene.

fresh figs with ricotta cheese and parma ham

1 Cut the figs into 4, leaving them attached at the base.

2 Stir the ricotta with the mustard and season to taste with salt and pepper.

3 Divide the ricotta mixture between the figs, spooning it over the top. Place two figs on each serving plate and top with some Parma ham.

4 Drizzle over the balsamic vinegar and serve the figs with crusty bread.

8 fresh figs

125 g (4 oz) ricotta cheese

1 teaspoon Dijon mustard

85 g (3¼ oz) Parma ham

2 tablespoons balsamic vinegar

salt and pepper

crusty bread, to serve

NUTRITIONAL FACTS

GI rating: LOW

- Kcals – 139
- Protein – 10 g
- Carbohydrate – 11 g
- Fat – 6 g

NUTRITIONAL TIP

Both fresh figs and dried figs are a good source of antioxidant vitamins, fibre and potassium.

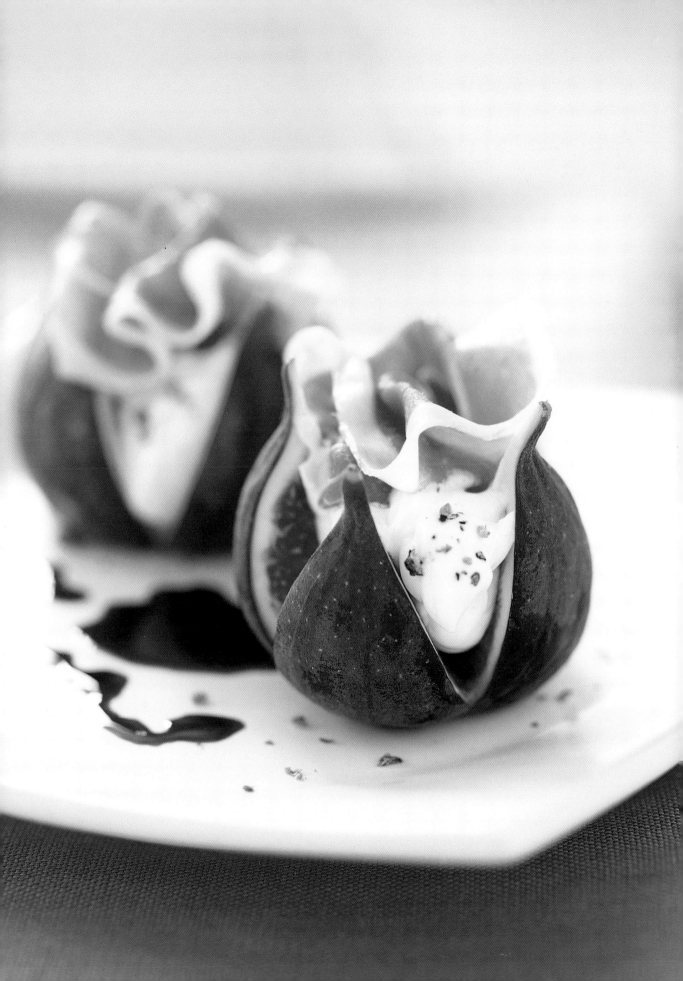

vegetable curry

1 tablespoon olive oil

1 onion, chopped

1 garlic clove, crushed

2 tablespoons medium curry paste

1½ kg (3 lb) prepared mixed vegetables
   (such as courgette, pepper, squash,
   mushrooms and green beans)

200 g (7 oz) can chopped tomatoes

400 g (13 oz) can reduced fat coconut
   milk

2 tablespoons chopped coriander
   leaves

boiled rice, to serve

1 Heat the oil in a large saucepan, add the onion and garlic and fry for 2 minutes. Stir in the curry paste and fry for 1 minute more.

2 Add the vegetables and fry for 2–3 minutes, stirring occasionally, then add the tomatoes and coconut milk. Stir well, bring to the boil, then lower the heat and simmer for 12–15 minutes until all the vegetables are cooked.

3 Stir in the coriander and serve with rice.

NUTRITIONAL FACTS

 Suitable for vegetarians

GI rating: MEDIUM

- Kcals – 172
- Protein – 6 g
- Carbohydrate – 26 g
- Fat – 5 g

NUTRITIONAL TIP

Transform this vegetable curry into a well-balanced meal with the addition of rice and an Indian bread.

baked red fruits with crispy topping

1 kg (2 lb) mixed summer berries
    (such as strawberries, raspberries
    and blackberries)
grated rind and juice of 1 orange

TOPPING
75 g (3 oz) crunchy oat cereal
75 g (3 oz) porridge oats
25 g (1 oz) melted butter
1 tablespoon clear honey
25 g (1 oz) chopped hazelnuts

1 Place the fruits, orange rind and juice in an ovenproof dish.

2 Cook in a preheated oven at 200°C (400°F), Gas Mark 6, for 10 minutes until the juices begin to run.

3 Mix together all the topping ingredients and sprinkle over the fruits.

4 Return the dish to the oven and cook for a further 10 minutes until bubbling and golden on top.

NUTRITIONAL FACTS

 Suitable for vegetarians

GI rating: MEDIUM

- Kcals – 331
- Protein – 8 g
- Carbohydrate – 50 g
- Fat – 12 g

NUTRITIONAL TIP

Porridge oats are high in soluble fibre and have a low glycaemic index. Porridge is a useful snack food.

griddled pineapple and ginger

2 tablespoons icing sugar

1 teaspoon ground ginger

1 pineapple, peeled and cut into 2.5 cm (1 inch) thick rounds

4 tablespoons virtually fat-free fromage frais, to serve

1 Heat a griddle or a heavy-based frying pan until hot.

2 Mix together the icing sugar and ginger and sprinkle over both sides of the pineapple rings. Place the pineapple on the griddle and cook for 1–2 minutes on each side until golden.

3 Serve the pineapple hot with the fromage frais.

NUTRITIONAL FACTS

 Suitable for vegetarians

GI rating: MEDIUM–HIGH

- Kcals – 107
- Protein – 4 g
- Carbohydrate – 23 g
- Fat – 0

NUTRITIONAL TIP

Pineapple contains bromelain, an enzyme which breaks down protein.

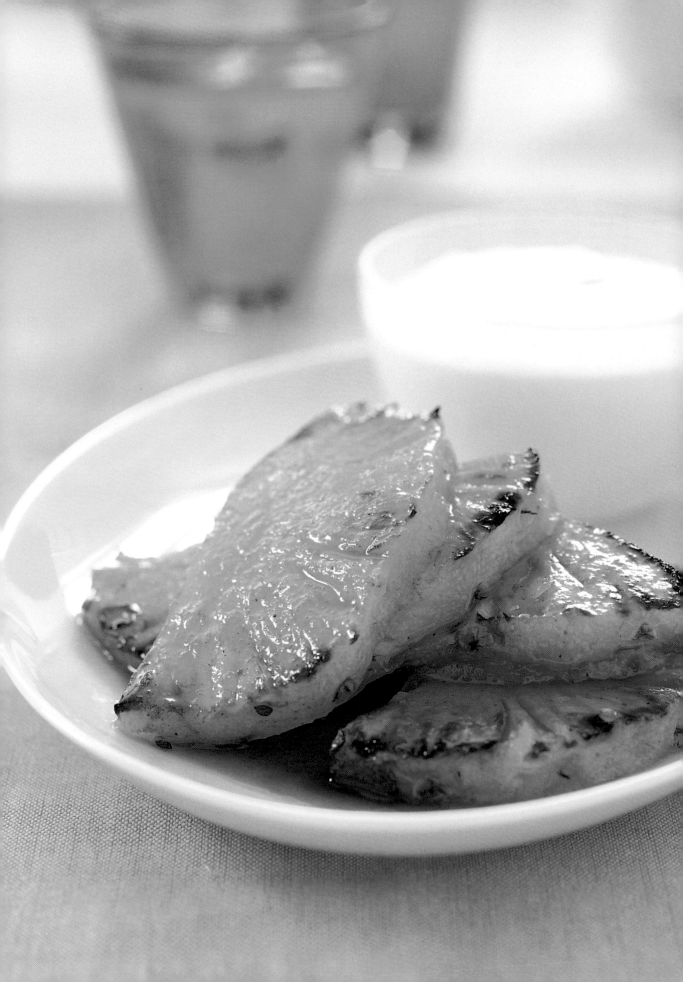

tropical fruit salad

1 Combine all the ingredients in a large serving bowl, cover and leave in the refrigerator for 20 minutes for the flavours to develop.

1 melon, deseeded and cubed

425 g (14 oz) can pineapple cubes in natural juice, drained and juice reserved

2 kiwifruits, sliced

1 papaya, cubed

4 tablespoons lime juice

2 pieces preserved ginger in syrup, finely chopped, plus 2 tablespoons of the syrup

pulp and seeds of 2 passion fruits

NUTRITIONAL FACTS

 Suitable for vegetarians

GI rating: MEDIUM–HIGH

- Kcals – 94
- Protein – 2 g
- Carbohydrate – 22 g
- Fat – 0 g

NUTRITIONAL TIP

One kiwifruit contains the recommended daily allowance of vitamin C.

watermelon granita

1 Place all the ingredients in a food processor or blender and blend until smooth.

2 Serve immediately in frosted glasses.

1 watermelon, deseeded, cubed and
   frozen
grated rind and juice of 1 lime
2 tablespoons icing sugar

NUTRITIONAL FACTS

 Suitable for vegetarians

   GI rating: HIGH

- Kcals – 92
- Protein – 1 g
- Carbohydrate – 22 g
- Fat – 1 g

NUTRITIONAL TIP

To reduce the sugar in this recipe use granulated intense sweetener instead.

individual lime and raspberry cheesecakes

6 ginger biscuits, lightly crushed

200 g (7 oz) extra-light cream cheese

200 g (7 oz) virtually fat-free
   fromage frais

few drops of vanilla extract

1 tablespoon caster sugar

grated rind and juice of 1 lime

125 g (4 oz) raspberries

lime wedges, to garnish

1 Divide the biscuits between 4 small glass dishes.

2 In a bowl, mix together the cream cheese, fromage frais, vanilla extract, sugar, and lime rind and juice.

3 Spoon the mixture on to the biscuits, then top with the raspberries. Serve immediately garnished with a lime wedge.

NUTRITIONAL FACTS

 Suitable for vegetarians

GI rating: MEDIUM–HIGH

- Kcals – 180
- Protein – 8 g
- Carbohydrate – 23 g
- Fat – 7 g

NUTRITIONAL TIP

Choose very fresh raspberries as they have a higher antioxidant content and are more nutritious.

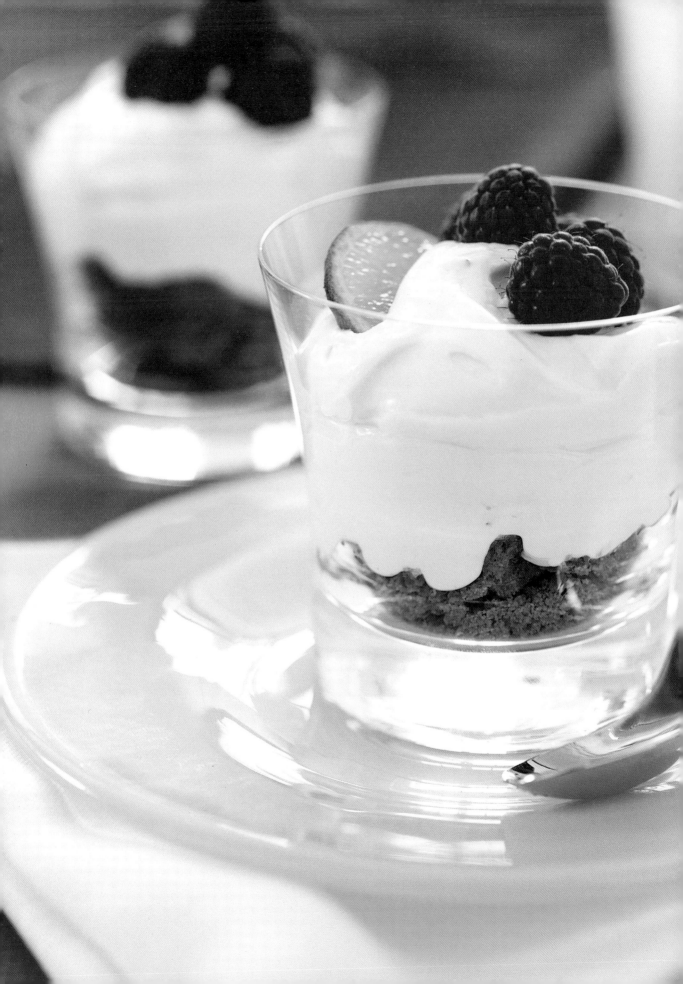

grilled nectarines with mint vanilla cream

1 Place the nectarines on a grill pan, cut side up. Mix together the cinnamon, honey and orange rind and juice, and drizzle over the nectarines.

2 Place the nectarines under a preheated hot grill and cook for 7–8 minutes, until golden, basting occasionally with the juices.

3 Mix together the crème fraîche, yogurt, mint and vanilla extract and serve with the nectarines.

4 nectarines, halved and stoned

pinch of ground cinnamon

1 tablespoon clear honey

grated rind and juice of 1 orange

4 tablespoons light crème fraîche

150 g (5 oz) natural yogurt

1 tablespoon chopped mint

few drops of vanilla extract

NUTRITIONAL FACTS

 Suitable for vegetarians

GI rating: MEDIUM

○ Kcals – 108

○ Protein – 4 g

○ Carbohydrate – 23 g

○ Fat – 3 g

NUTRITIONAL TIP

Natural yogurt is low in fat and can be used in sweet and savoury dishes.

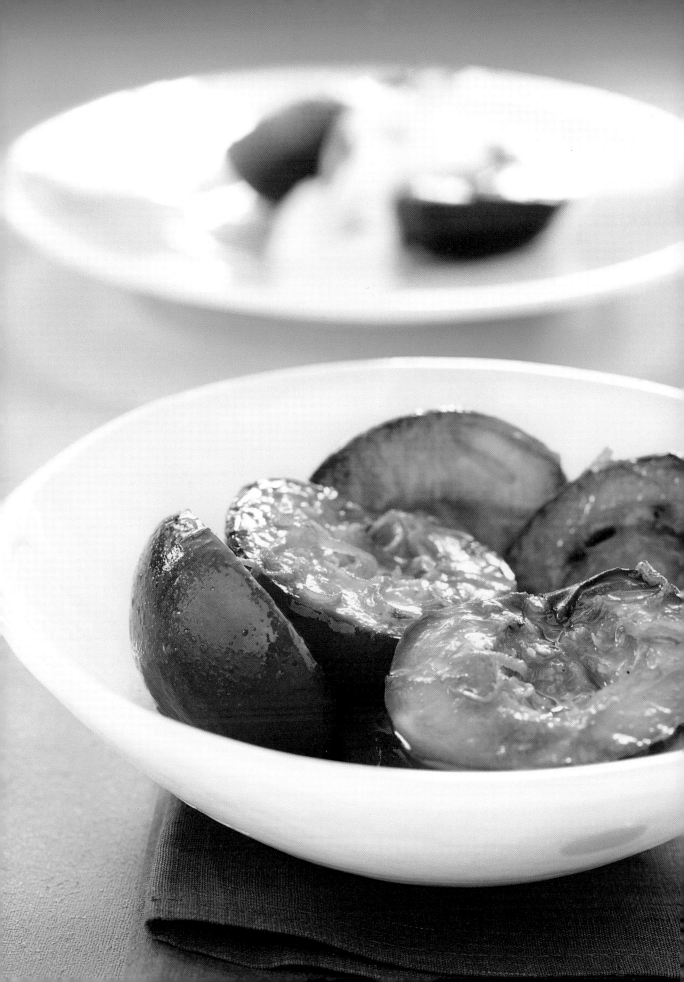

super smoothies

1 Place all the ingredients in a food processor or blender and blend until smooth.

2 Serve in tall glasses.

STRAWBERRY

1 banana, chopped

500 g (1 lb) strawberries, hulled

900 ml (1½ pints) ice-cold
   semi-skimmed milk

PEACH MELBA

1 banana, chopped

2 peaches, stoned

250 g (8 oz) strawberries, hulled

900 ml (1½ pints) ice-cold
   semi-skimmed milk

TROPICAL

500 g (1 lb) frozen tropical fruits, almost
   defrosted

600 ml (1 pint) ice-cold unsweetened
   pineapple juice

strawberry	peach melba	tropical
● Kcals –158	● Kcals – 159	● Kcals – 105
● Protein – 9 g	● Protein – 9 g	● Protein – 1 g
● Carbohydrate – 25 g	● Carbohydrate – 25 g	● Carbohydrate – 27 g
● Fat – 3 g	● Fat – 3 g	● Fat – 0 g

NUTRITIONAL TIP

Smoothies are packed with vitamins and fibre and a good way of consuming the recommended daily allowance of fruit.

NUTRITIONAL FACTS

 Suitable for vegetarians

GI rating: MEDIUM

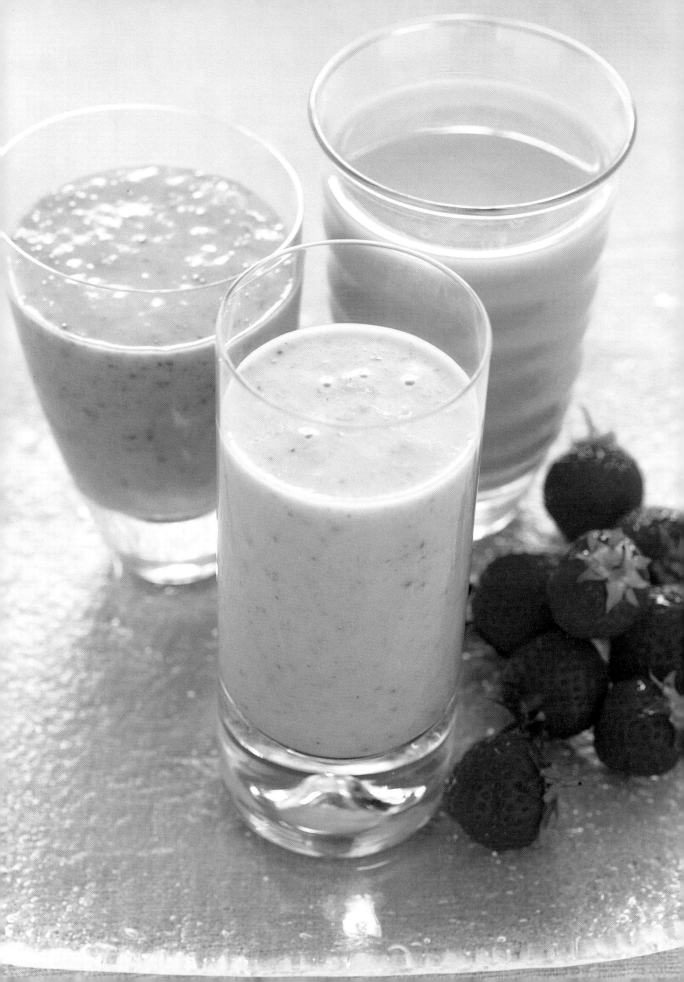

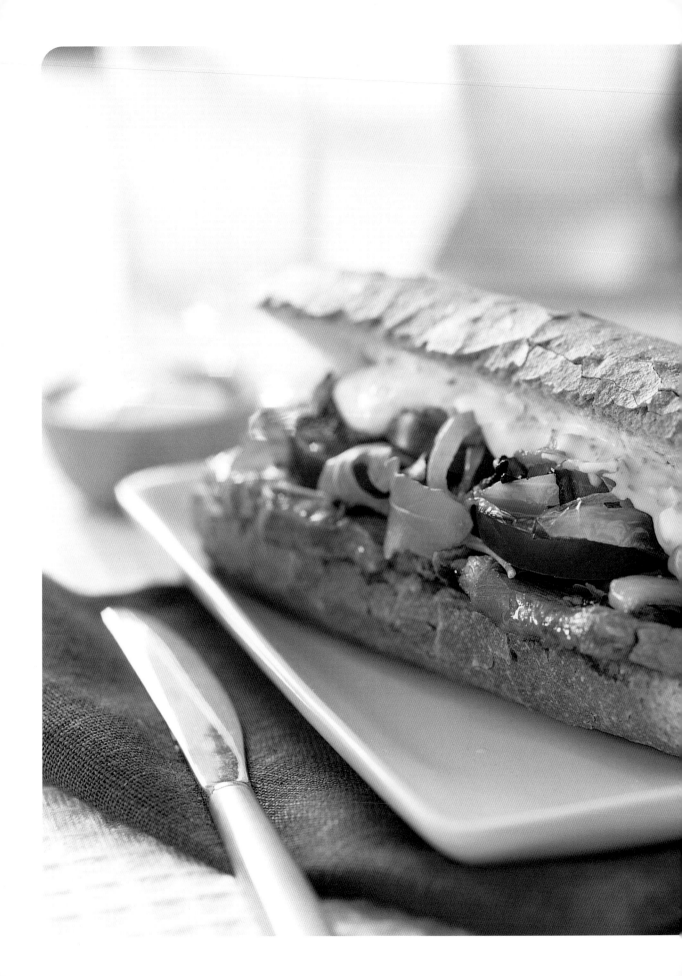

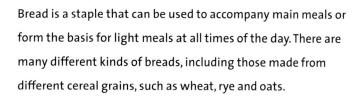

bread
as a basis

Bread is a staple that can be used to accompany main meals or form the basis for light meals at all times of the day. There are many different kinds of breads, including those made from different cereal grains, such as wheat, rye and oats.

There are also wholegrain breads, and breads made from processed cereals, producing a lower-fibre, white bread. Pumpernickel bread is made from rye kernels and has a low glycaemic index compared to breads made from wheat flours (wholemeal or refined). Multigrain breads and bread with added fruit has a lower glycaemic index than standard white and wholemeal loaves.

Whichever bread you choose, it can help to increase the carbohydrate content of a meal and provide a healthy balance. Try some of the recipes for muffins and other baked foods which you can use to add variety to your diet. These can be as convenient and delicious as simply slicing a loaf.

baked tortillas with hummus

1 Cut each tortilla into 8 triangles, place on a baking sheet and brush with a little oil. Place in a preheated oven at 200°C (400°F), Gas Mark 6, and bake for 10–12 minutes until golden and crisp. Leave to cool.

2 Meanwhile, put all the ingredients for the hummus, except the paprika and coriander, in a food processor or blender and blend until almost smooth. Season to taste with salt and pepper, stir in the coriander and sprinkle with paprika. Garnish with a coriander sprig and serve with the tortilla chips.

4 small flour tortillas
1 tablespoon olive oil

HUMMUS
400 g (13 oz) can chickpeas, drained
    and rinsed
1 garlic clove
4 tablespoons Greek yogurt
2 tablespoons lemon juice
1 tablespoon chopped coriander leaves
salt and pepper
paprika, to serve
coriander sprig, to garnish

NUTRITIONAL FACTS

 Suitable for vegetarians

GI rating: LOW

- Kcals – 306
- Protein – 12 g
- Carbohydrate – 46 g
- Fat – 9 g

NUTRITIONAL TIP

Shop-bought tortilla chips and hummus are high in fat. This recipe is a delicious low-fat alternative.

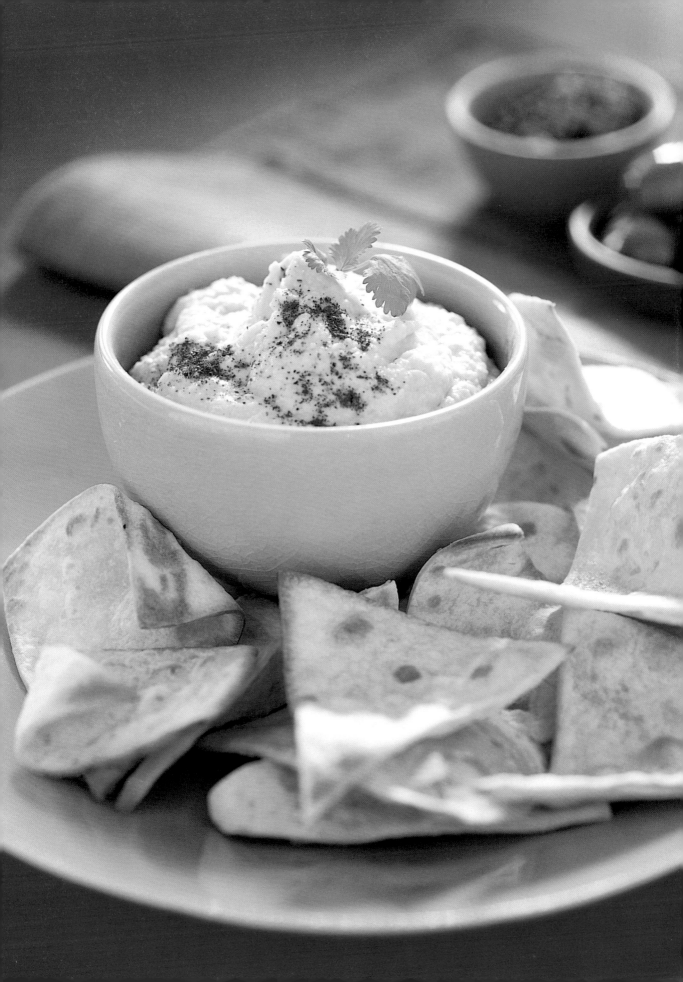

pitta with citrus chicken brochettes

3 boneless, skinless chicken
  breasts, cubed
1 teaspoon chopped thyme
grated rind and juice of 1 orange
grated rind and juice of 1 lime
1 red pepper, cored, deseeded
  and cubed
1 onion, cut into wedges
4 large pitta breads
60 g (2½ oz) salad leaves
4 tablespoons Greek yogurt
1 tablespoon chopped mint

1 Place the chicken cubes in a non-metallic dish with the thyme, and orange and lemon rinds and juice, and leave to marinate for 10 minutes.

2 Divide the chicken, red pepper and onion between 8 wooden barbecue skewers.

3 Place the brochettes under a preheated moderate grill for 7–8 minutes, turning occasionally and brushing with a little marinade from time to time, until browned and cooked through.

4 Warm the pittas and slit along one side to make a pocket. Fill with the salad leaves and the brochettes.

5 Mix together the yogurt and mint and spoon into the pittas. Serve hot.

NUTRITIONAL FACTS

GI rating: MEDIUM

- Kcals – 437
- Protein – 42 g
- Carbohydrate – 53 g
- Fat – 7 g

NUTRITIONAL TIP

Served with plenty of salad, these pittas are a complete meal.

italian
bread salad

1 Put the bread on a grill pan in one layer, place under a preheated moderate grill and toast until golden all over.

2 In a large bowl, mix the bread with tomatoes, cucumber, capers, red onion, olives, basil and French dressing. Season with black pepper and set aside for 10 minutes to allow the flavours to develop. Serve at room temperature.

1 ciabatta loaf, torn into
   bite-sized pieces
4 tomatoes, cut into chunks
½ cucumber, chopped
3 tablespoons capers, drained
1 red onion, finely sliced
24 black olives, pitted
handful of basil, torn
4 tablespoons virtually fat-free
   French dressing
black pepper

NUTRITIONAL FACTS

 Suitable for vegetarians

   GI rating: MEDIUM

- Kcals – 236
- Protein – 8 g
- Carbohydrate – 44 g
- Fat – 4 g

NUTRITIONAL TIP

Olives contain natural antioxidants called polyphenols, they are also a good source of vitamin E.

steak sandwiches

1 Heat a griddle or nonstick frying pan until very hot.

2 Place the steak on the griddle and cook for 2 minutes on each side, or until cooked to taste. Remove the steak and leave it to rest for 5 minutes.

3 Meanwhile, add the oil to the griddle and fry the onion for 2–3 minutes.

4 Mix together the crème fraîche and mustard.

5 Assemble the sandwich by placing the steak in the bread, then add the rocket, tomato and onion. Finish with a dollop of the mustard and crème fraîche mixture and season to taste with salt and pepper.

4 pieces thin cut sirloin steak, about 125 g (4 oz) each

1 tablespoon oil

1 onion, sliced

4 tablespoons light crème fraîche

1 tablespoon wholegrain mustard

1 French stick, cut into 4 and split down one side

60 g (2½ oz) rocket

2 tomatoes, sliced

salt and pepper

NUTRITIONAL FACTS

GI rating: MEDIUM
- Kcals – 388
- Protein – 30 g
- Carbohydrate – 46 g
- Fat – 12 g

NUTRITIONAL TIP

Lean steak is full of nutrients and minerals, it is also a low fat sandwich filling.

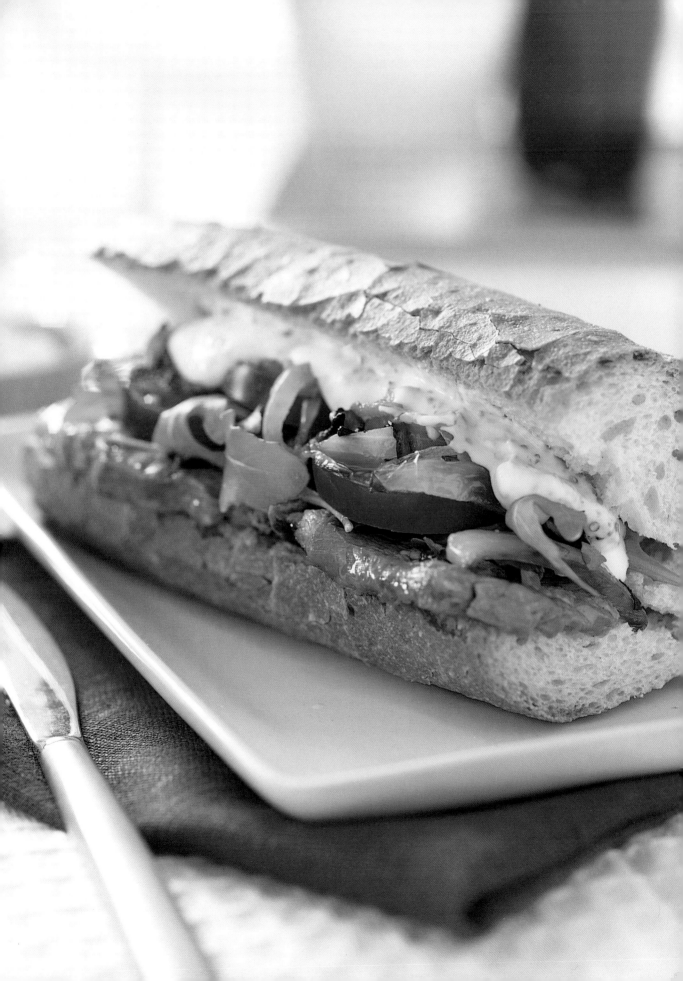

tasty open toasties

4 thick slices of granary bread

4 slices of lean ham

2 tomatoes, sliced

4 eggs

1 tablespoon white wine vinegar

3 tablespoons light crème fraîche

2 tablespoons chopped herbs (such as
  parsley or tarragon)

salt and pepper

1 Toast the bread on both sides, then top each piece with a slice of ham and 2 tomato slices.

2 To poach the eggs, bring a large saucepan of water to the boil, add the vinegar, then stir the water rapidly in a circular motion to create a whirlpool. Break an egg into the centre of the pan to allow the white to wrap around the yolk. Cook for 3 minutes then remove from the pan and keep warm. Repeat with the remaining eggs, then place 1 egg on each piece of toast.

3 Mix together the crème fraîche and herbs, season to taste with salt and pepper and serve with the toasties.

NUTRITIONAL FACTS

GI rating: MEDIUM

- Kcals – 212
- Protein – 14 g
- Carbohydrate – 21 g
- Fat – 11 g

NUTRITIONAL TIP

Granary bread has additional wholewheat grains added to the mixture, making it rougher in texture and lower in glycaemic index.

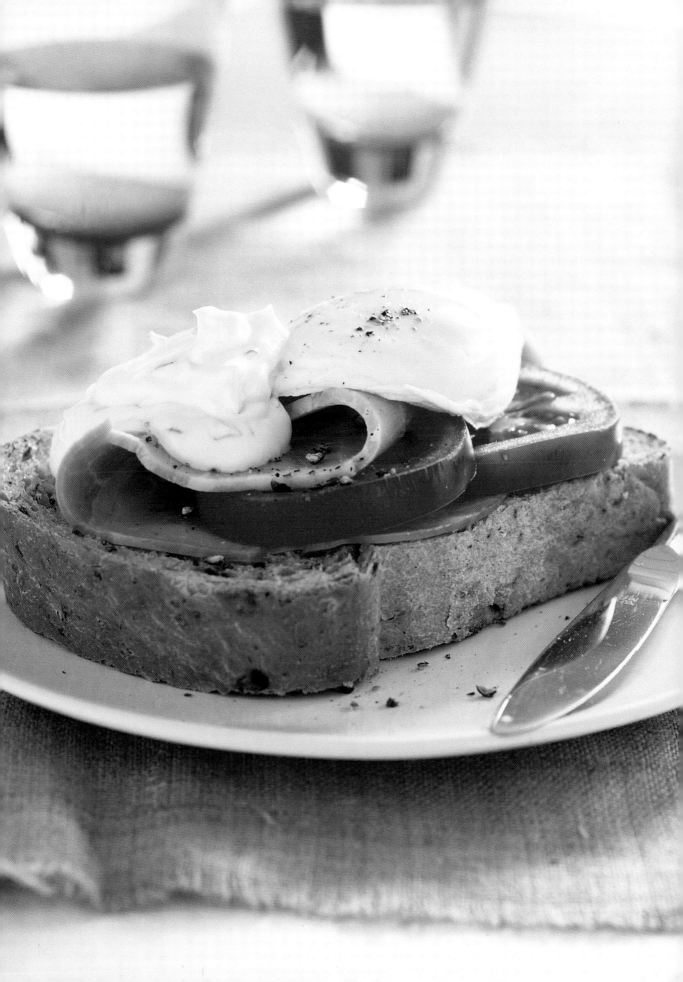

mixed open sandwiches

1 To make blue cheese and pear open sandwiches, simply divide the ingredients between 4 slices of bread and drizzle with balsamic vinegar.

2 To make Thai prawn open sandwiches, stir all the ingredients together and divide between the slices of bread.

3 To make the Mediterranean topping, divide the peppers and artichoke hearts between the bread, drizzle over the oil and sprinkle over the torn basil.

12 slices of mixed breads, to serve

BLUE CHEESE AND PEAR

1 bunch of watercress, roughly chopped

1 large ripe pear, cored and sliced

50 g (2 oz) blue cheese
   (such as Stilton), sliced

2 teaspoons balsamic vinegar

THAI PRAWN

200 g (7 oz) extra-light cream cheese

grated rind and juice of ½ lime

100 g (3½ oz) cooked peeled prawns,
   roughly chopped

2 tablespoons chopped coriander
   leaves

MEDITERRANEAN

2 red peppers, roasted and sliced

4 artichoke hearts in oil, drained
   and quartered

1 tablespoon olive oil

2 tablespoons torn basil

blue cheese
- Kcals –221
- Protein – 8g
- Carbohydrate – 36 g
- Fat – 6g

thai prawn
- Kcals – 177
- Protein – 10 g
- Carbohydrate – 23 g
- Fat – 5 g

mediterranean
- Kcals – 173
- Protein – 6 g
- Carbohydrate – 29g
- Fat – 5g

NUTRITIONAL TIP
Red peppers are a good source of carotenoids, thought to preserve health, and also vitamin C.

NUTRITIONAL FACTS
GI rating: LOW–MEDIUM

mozzarella burgers

500 g (1 lb) extra-lean minced beef

1 small onion, finely chopped

pinch of paprika

1 egg, beaten

2 tablespoons chopped parsley

70 g (2 ¾ oz) mozzarella cheese, cut
   into 4 slices

4 large baps or small ciabatta rolls

1 red pepper, roasted, skinned,
   deseeded and sliced

12 basil leaves

60 g (2½ oz) salad leaves

salt and pepper

1 Place the mince, onion, paprika and egg into a food processor or blender and blend until well combined. Season with salt and pepper, then stir in the parsley and divide the mixture into 4 pieces.

2 Mould each piece of meat mixture around a piece of mozzarella, to completely enclose the cheese and make a burger shape.

3 Place the burgers under a preheated hot grill or on a barbecue for 8–10 minutes, turning halfway through cooking, until browned on both sides and cooked through.

4 Serve the burgers in the baps, topped with roasted pepper slices, basil and salad leaves.

NUTRITIONAL FACTS

GI rating: LOW

- Kcals – 429
- Protein – 37 g
- Carbohydrate – 29 g
- Fat – 17 g

NUTRITIONAL TIP

Use half-fat mozzarella cheese to cut down on fat.

chicken fajitas

1 Heat the oil in a frying pan, add the chicken and fry for 2–3 minutes until beginning to brown.

2 Add the onions, peppers and chilli flakes and continue to fry for 5 minutes more. Remove from the heat and stir in the coriander and lime juice.

3 Warm the tortillas according to the packet instructions, then fill them with the chicken mixture and crème fraîche, garnish with coriander sprigs and serve.

1 tablespoon olive oil

2 boneless, skinless chicken breasts, sliced

2 red onions, cut into wedges

2 red peppers, cored, deseeded and sliced

1 yellow pepper, cored, deseeded and sliced

pinch of dried chilli flakes

2 tablespoons chopped coriander leaves

2 tablespoons lime juice

8 medium flour tortillas

4 tablespoons light crème fraîche

60 g (2½ oz) salad leaves, to serve

NUTRITIONAL FACTS

GI rating: MEDIUM

- Kcals – 328
- Protein – 26 g
- Carbohydrate – 46 g
- Fat – 7 g

NUTRITIONAL TIP

Chicken is full of vitamins and minerals and with the skin removed it is also low in fat.

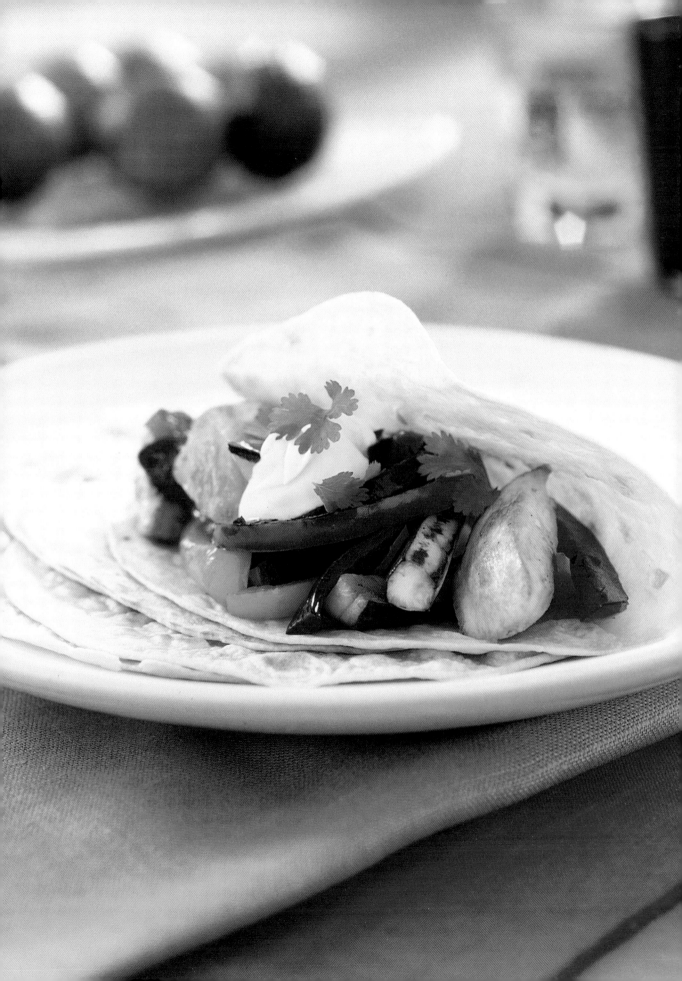

grilled chicken sandwich

1 Heat the oil in a nonstick frying pan, add the onion and fry for 2–3 minutes, until beginning to soften.

2 Add the chicken to the pan and continue to fry for 4–5 minutes, until the chicken is browned and cooked through. Stir in the yogurt and season well with black pepper.

3 Fill the bread with the chicken and rocket and serve.

1 tablespoon oil

1 onion, sliced

2 boneless, skinless chicken breasts, sliced

2 tablespoons natural yogurt

1 French stick, quartered and split along one side

60 g (2½ oz) rocket

salt and pepper

NUTRITIONAL FACTS

GI rating: MEDIUM

- Kcals – 256
- Protein – 26 g
- Carbohydrate – 27 g
- Fat – 5 g

NUTRITIONAL TIP

Always remove the skin from chicken before cooking to reduce the fat content.

smoked haddock and poached egg muffins

1 Place the fish in a large frying pan, pour over the milk and add the bay leaf and peppercorns. Bring to the boil, then simmer gently for 4–5 minutes, until the fish is just cooked.

2 Bring another pan of water to the boil and add the vinegar. Stir the water rapidly in a circular motion to create a whirlpool. Break an egg into the centre of the pan to allow the white to wrap around the yolk. Cook for 3 minutes then remove from the pan and keep warm. Repeat with the remaining eggs.

3 Place a few rocket leaves on the bottom half of each muffin, and top with a piece of fish and a poached egg.

4 Spoon over the hollandaise, sprinkle with pepper and serve topped with the other muffin half.

4 pieces skinless, natural smoked haddock, about 100 g (3½ oz) each

300 ml (½ pint) milk

1 bay leaf

2 peppercorns

1 tablespoon white wine vinegar

4 eggs

60 g (2½ oz) rocket

4 breakfast muffins, halved and toasted

4 tablespoons reduced-fat hollandaise sauce

pepper

NUTRITIONAL FACTS

GI rating: MEDIUM–HIGH

- Kcals – 433
- Protein – 36 g
- Carbohydrate – 39 g
- Fat – 14 g

NUTRITIONAL TIP

Smoked haddock is high in sodium but cooking it in a liquid such as milk helps to reduce the sodium content.

smoked salmon blinis with dill cream

1 Gently warm the blinis for a few minutes under a grill or in the oven.

2 Stir together the crème fraîche, dill, lemon rind and spring onions and season with pepper. Spoon the mixture on to the blinis and top with the salmon. Garnish with lemon wedges and serve.

8 large blinis

2 tablespoons light crème fraîche

1 teaspoon chopped dill

grated rind of 1 lemon

2 spring onions, sliced

100 g (3½ oz) smoked salmon

lemon wedges, to garnish

pepper

NUTRITIONAL FACTS

GI rating: MEDIUM

- Kcals – 171
- Protein – 9 g
- Carbohydrate – 20 g
- Fat – 8 g

NUTRITIONAL TIP

Light crème fraîche is lower in fat than single cream and has only a third of the fat of standard crème fraîche.